Foundations of Exercise and Mental Health

Larry M. Leith, Ph.D.
University of Toronto

FITNESS INFORMATION TECHNOLOGY, INC.
P.O. BOX 4425, UNIVERSITY AVE.
MORGANTOWN, WV 26504

The exercises, psychological interventions, and
assessments recommended
in this book should be performed by individuals
with appropriate training
and credentials. The exercises prescribed are not
intended for use by the
general public without
appropriate evaluation and
supervision by certified
exercise specialists.

Front cover photo courtesy
of HealthWorks, Inc.,
Morgantown, WV.
Reprinted with permission.

LOC: 01-135398
ISBN: 1-885693-41-9

Cover Design: Bellerophon Productions
Copyeditor: Sandra R. Woods

Printed in the United States of America
10 9 8 7 6 5 4 3

Fitness Information Technology, Inc.
P.O. Box 4425
University Avenue
Morgantown, WV 26504
800.477.4348
304.599.3483
304.599.3482 (fax)

Table of Contents

Acknowledgments

There are many people to thank for their support and technical advice during the writing of this book. First, my wife, Nancy, for putting up with the long hours I spent on the word processor --thanks for your understanding and support. I also benefited greatly from an initial review of the manuscript by Dr. Brent Rushall at San Diego State University. I would like to thank Dr. John Raglin at Indiana University-Bloomington and Dr. Wesley Sime at the University of Nebraska for their critical reviews of the final product. Both of these individuals spent many hours reviewing the work and offering suggestions to make the book as comprehensive as possible. I also appreciate their positive approach. In terms of exercise assessment and prescription, I received excellent advice from two colleagues at the University of Toronto. Karen Lewis was helpful in recommending appropriate field tests for exercise assessment. In addition, Dr. Jack Goodman's advice was invaluable in the development and critical review of chapter 7. His state-of-the-art knowledge of exercise assessment and prescription was instrumental in the completion of this product. Finally, my sincere thanks to Dr. Andrew Ostrow and Fitness Information Technology, Inc., for believing in the product and helping me complete a lifelong goal.

Foreword

My primary training has been in medicine and in physiology, but like many of my colleagues I have always had a fascination with the workings of the human mind, and on a number of occasions-- both the colleagues trained in psychology, and (more adventurously!) without such assistance, I have undertaken studies examining the determinants of exercise behaviour, and the impact of physical activity upon mental health in sport, in industry and in disease. I was thus very excited when I learned that Dr. Larry Leith was preparing a monograph that would provide an in-depth exploration of the inter-relationships between regular exercise and mental health.

As will be plain from the content, Dr. Leith writes from extensive personal experience, gained both in graduate and undergraduate teaching and research studies, including a recent detailed literature search undertaken on behalf of the Canadian government. Confidence in the volume is further enhanced by the detailed review that the manuscript has received from several of the other giants in this area of knowledge. The academic and graduate student will be particularly attracted by the clear tables setting out and summarizing the currently available research knowledge on individual topics, and the mental health practitioner will be equally attracted by the clear recommendations for exercise programs to address each of the major problem areas of mental health.

I have known Dr. Leith for some 14 years now, having recognized his ability and recruited him to the School of Physical and Health Education at the University of Toronto in my early period of faculty building as Director of that institution. I was immediately impressed, not only by his intellectual ability and range of knowledge, but also by the strength of his own mental health. His self-image was sufficiently good that he was prepared to leave a tenured appointment elsewhere for a vacancy that (in Toronto) was initially untenured, and throughout his 14 years in Toronto he has consistently demonstrated a good humour and cheerfulness in the face of both the joys and the inevitable disappointments of life; plainly, he has been able to put his store of knowledge to tremendous personal use, and the practical techniques he suggests are methods that work! His teaching record has been equally impressive, and I was quickly astonished by his ability to address each of a class of 140 students by their first names within the first two weeks of term. This excellent rapport allowed a real dialogue with class members, again helpful to the preparation of this monograph, and reflected also in a number of prestigious teaching awards.

This is not the first book that Dr. Leith has written, and he is still sufficiently young and energetic that it will not be the last. Nevertheless, "Foundations of Exercise and Mental Health" will be recognized as one of Larry's important contributions to our understanding and practice of exercise psychology, and I would warmly commend this book to all with an interest in mental health, whether exercise scientists, mental health practitioners or family physicians.

Toronto, July 1994.   Roy J. Shephard, M.D., Ph.D., D.P.E.

Preface

The idea for this book evolved as a result of lifelong interests in the academic disciplines of psychology and physical education. As an undergraduate, then graduate physical education student, I filled my electives with the maximum number of psychology courses allowed. Although it would be ego-gratifying to claim a perceived need for this marriage of disciplines, the reality of the matter was that I simply liked both subjects equally. Today, I still do. This book is an attempt to consummate the marriage between psychology and physical education as they relate to areas of personal interest.

Foundations of Exercise and Mental Health is written for all individuals interested in the effect of exercise on psychological and emotional well-being. Three particular subgroups will find the book to be of particular value. First, exercise scientists and their graduate students will find the information timely from both a classroom and a research perspective. From an educational standpoint, this publication provides justification for the long-term promotion of an active life-style among both student and adult populations. The collated research provides direction and focus for future investigations in this area. A second interest group involves mental health practitioners, such as counsellors, psychologists, and psychiatrists. The increasing use of exercise as a practical form of therapy highlights the need for information concerning appropriate and specific exercise intervention strategies. This book thus serves as a valuable resource for mental health practitioners seeking this important information. A final interest group includes medical practitioners, particularly family physicians. Many doctors are now recognizing the importance of an active life-style to both physical and mental health. The medical practitioner who adopts a holistic approach to health will find this publication to be of special value.

Research investigating the exercise and mental health relationship has evolved as a series of unrelated experiments attempting to relate the effects of a specific exercise on a specific psychological construct in a specific sample. This publication expands current knowledge by integrating and synthesizing the findings from these isolated and varied empirical research studies into meaningful conclusions. In addition, the appropriateness of specific exercises for specific psychological benefits is fully discussed.

This book is an introduction to the expanding field of exercise and mental health. I begin by providing an overview of the prevalence of mental disorders in modern society, illustrate the evolution of research in this area, then provide some hypotheses with potential to explain the exercise and mental health relationship. Chapters 2 through 6 examine the effects of exercise on depression, anxiety, self-concept/self-esteem, personality, and mood. Each of these chapters includes a summary table of all empirical research investigating the topic. These tables are intended to provide an excellent reference for the researcher and practitioner alike. In addition, each chapter includes several exercise "Prescription Guidelines," inserted at appropriate points to highlight specific recommendations for prescribing exercise for the psychological construct under consideration. In each case, the prescription guideline is gleaned from, and immediately follows, the related research synthesis. Chapter 7 thoroughly examines current knowledge regarding exercise prescription. This chapter will prove especially valuable for the two target groups that have had limited exposure to the exercise process. This section of the text has been reviewed by an expert in the field of exercise assessment and prescription to insure that the exercises are both appropriate and safe for the participant. Finally, chapter 8 provides a general overview of the efficacy of exercise in promoting mental health and suggests directions for future research.

It has been satisfying to see the domain of exercise psychology become a frequent topic of symposia and original research presentations at national and international sports science conferences. It has also become an increasingly popular topic for graduate student research. The interest expressed in this area by students, exercise scientists, and medical professionals alike appears to be growing exponentially. *Foundations of Exercise and Mental Health* thus fills an important and timely need.

Chapter 1

INTRODUCTION

Mental health problems are pandemic in modern society. A landmark study from NIMH, the National Institute of Mental Health (Regier, et al., 1984) provides a comprehensive picture of mental illness in America. The $15-million investigation individually interviewed more than 17,000 people in five communities. As a source of diagnostic categories, the interviewers used the *Diagnostic and Statistical Manual of Mental Disorders* (American Psychiatric Association, 1980). A major finding of the NIMH study indicated that during a 6-month span, 20% (29 million) of the adult population experienced some form of mental disturbance, and it has been estimated that 29% to 38% of American adults can expect a significant psychiatric problem sometime during their lifetimes (Robins et al., 1984). However, only one in five of these individuals will seek professional help, usually in the form of a family physician rather than a psychiatrist (Shapiro et al., 1984). A more recent study confirms these findings, reporting the one-month prevalence rate of mental disorders in the United States to be 15.4%, with stress-related symptoms, such as anxiety and depression, accounting for the highest proportion of disorders (Regier et al., 1988). Stress has been estimated to be a factor in up to 50% of all visits to medical practitioners (Kuyler & Dunner, 1976). Traditionally, mental health problems such as these have been treated by psychotherapy and/or psychotropic medication. Although both techniques have merit, psychotherapy involves a relatively long time commitment, and psychotropic medications are often associated with a host of adverse side effects. For this reason, increasing interest has been paid to the use of alternative means of treating and preventing mental health problems. One such nontraditional technique involves the use of long-term, or chronic, exercise programs. The purpose of this book is to thoroughly examine the potential of exercise to impact positively on the mental health of the participant.

The objectives of this chapter are to (a) indicate the scope of mental health problems in society, (b) introduce the role of exercise in holistic health, (c) provide an historical overview of research in this important area, (d) suggest the value of exercise as a preventative and treatment intervention technique, and (e) develop the conceptual framework for the exercise and mental health relationship.

Exercise as a Health Behavior

Civilization has progressed through a number of evolutionary periods that have all had some effect on human health (Blair, 1988). The first major revolution in health care was aimed at wiping out infectious disease. Improved sanitation, vaccines, and immunization programs provided the major thrust for health improvement. In the United States today, only 1% of the people who die before their 75th birthday die from infectious diseases (Mullen, 1986). A second revolution in health care involved efforts to eliminate degenerative diseases. There appears to have been some success in this regard as evidenced by the increase in longevity among the general population. However, two-thirds (67%) of all deaths in America are associated with diseases of old age (Illich, 1976). A third major revolution in health care has developed in a slow but systematic fashion throughout the world. This revolution has taken on different shapes and has been called different names. The overall goal of this new approach is maximum well-being or wellness. It puts emphasis on health rather than disease, with the process being long-term and preventive. It is in this third major revolution in health care that exercise is becoming recognized as having potential as a positive health behavior. Traditionally, the role of exercise on health was viewed predominantly from a biological or physiological perspective. Recently, however, the role of exercise in treating or preventing a variety of mental disorders has received increased attention. The evolution of exercise as a health behavior will now be briefly considered from both a physiological and psychological perspective.

Physiological Benefits of Exercise

From a physiological perspective, evidence indicates regular exercise has beneficial effects on such diverse areas as obstructive pulmonary disease management (Atkins, Kaplan, Timms, Reinsch, & Lofback, 1984), cardiovascular adaptation (Clausen, 1977; Fox & Haskell, 1978; Shephard, 1981), and obesity prevention and treatment (American College of Sports Medicine, 1983). Fragmentary evidence also suggests exercise may offer treatment for, and possible prevention of, hypertension (Seals & Hagberg, 1984), diabetes (Soman, Koivisto, Deibert, Felig, & DeFronze, 1979), and aging (Holloszy, 1983; Leith, 1982; Shephard & Leith, 1990; Spirduso, 1983). As a consequence of this accumulating evidence, exercise is slowly starting to be recognized as an important part of community medicine and public health policy. In the United States, the Department of Health and Human Services (1980) published national health objectives for the 1990s, with 11 of these objectives specifically referring to physical fitness and exercise (Powell, Spain, Christenson, & Mollenkamp, 1986). Traditionally, the effect of exercise on health has been viewed primarily from a physiological perspective, with attention focused largely on changes that take place in physiological functioning as the body becomes more physically fit. During the past decade, however, increasing attention has been focused on the psychological outcomes of exercise. The remainder of *Foundations of Exercise and Mental Health* will deal exclusively with this phenomenon.

Psychological Benefits of Exercise: An Historical Perspective

Hippocrates, often referred to as the father of medicine, reportedly prescribed exercise for patients suffering from mental illness (Ryan, 1984). In more recent times, however, the medical model of medicine and psychiatry promoted a more dualistic approach to physical and mental health. As a result, only the relatively small academic and professional schools of physical education, therapeutic recreation, and psychosomatic medicine maintained an interest in the relationship between exercise and mental health (Dishman, 1986). Fortunately, this situation has started to change.

The earliest pioneer empirical study can be traced to Franz and Hamilton (1905), who published a paper dealing with the effect of exercise in retarding depression. A review of related literature reveals that this study is seldom cited and appears to have minimal impact on the development of future studies. Since the first empirical investigation, research has continued to proliferate to the point of a well-referenced data base.

Prior to 1970, research investigating the exercise and mental health relationship continued to support the notion that positive psychological benefits could accrue from regular exercise. These early studies, however, must be viewed with caution due to several methodological problems associated with their research design (Cureton, 1963; Layman, 1960, 1972; Morgan, 1969,

1974, 1976, 1979a, 1981, 1982, 1985, 1988). Perhaps the best synopsis of the early empirical studies is provided by Morgan (1988), who suggests that (a) the early studies were based predominantly on correlational analyses and cross-section comparisons, (b) a causal relationship between psychopathology and fitness measures has not been established, and (c) even if a causal relationship had been documented, the results could not be generalized beyond the adult psychiatric patients studied in these experiments. Two additional observations concerning the early studies involve the fact that they employed global measures of mental health (e.g., personality, self-confidence) rather than specific constructs (e.g., depression, anxiety, mood) and utilized few females as sample populations (Layman, 1960, 1972). In spite of these methodological shortcomings, the majority of studies indicated that psychological benefits were associated with prolonged involvement in physical activity.

Recent research, especially those studies conducted from 1980 to present, have attempted to address the aforementioned problems. Major reviews by Doan and Scherman (1987), Folkins and Sime (1981), and Leith and Taylor (1990) have categorized empirical research on the bases of experimental designs. These reviews indicate a trend towards improved experimental rigor in recent research. They also reveal that more experiments are utilizing healthy sample populations, with an almost equal mix of male and female subjects. Even with the improved methodological rigor, the majority of studies still report that exercise is associated with significant psychological improvements in the participant. *Foundations of Exercise and Mental Health* will systematically review the nature of these psychological benefits.

The Mental Health/Mental Illness Distinction

Before engaging in a thorough review of the literature, it is important from both a theoretical and conceptual perspective to distinguish between mental health and mental illness. When we speak of mental illness, we are referring to individuals who are experiencing psychological problems of a clinical magnitude, with symptomology as categorized by the *Diagnostic and Statistical Manual of Mental Disorders* (American Psychiatric Association, 1987). In cases of this nature, the subjects are invariably under the treatment of a primary mental health care professional. Experiments involving this population utilize exercise as a form of treatment, or an adjunct to treatment, in an attempt to improve or eliminate the mental illness. In contrast, mental health categorizes those individuals who are not experiencing psychological problems of a clinical magnitude. Studies utilizing this population are concerned with the potential of exercise as a prevention strategy, or a form of health promotion. Although the early studies focused almost exclusively on the use of exercise as a form of treatment for mental problems, a trend has now developed that focuses on the potential of exercise to promote positive mental health. The conceptual framework emphasized throughout the remainder of this book maintains that exercise has the potential to impact positively on the mental health of all individuals, not merely those who are clinically symptomatic, as suggested by Morgan (1988). This suggested relationship is illustrated in Figure 1.1.

This representation illustrates how mental illness (point A) and mental health (point C) are part of the same continuum. When exercise is used as a form of treatment or therapy (treatment model), it has the potential to move an individual from point A to point B by alleviating the problematic psychological symptoms (e.g., anxiety, depression). This movement to the neutral point of the continuum represents the traditional goal of using exercise as therapy. When exercise is used as a form of health promotion (prevention model), it involves movement from point B toward point C on the continuum. The use of exercise in this manner represents a more recent line of research. An important implication that arises from Figure 1.1 is that we should not be content with merely eliminating clinical symptoms (a point A- to- point B move). This suggests when exercise is used as therapy, the

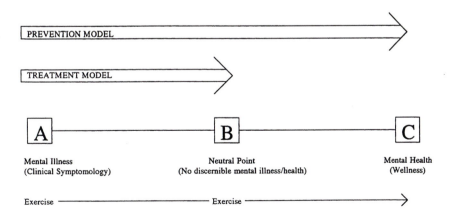

Figure 1.1. The exercise and mental health continuum, showing how exercise has the potential to act as both a treatment and a preventive measure.

goal should not merely be the absence of mental illness, but rather the attainment of mental health. All individuals, regardless of their initial starting point on the continuum, should strive toward mental health and not be content with the absence of clinical symptoms. Finally, because Figure 1.1 represents a continuum, it is important to remember that an individual's relative position on the continuum may vary from time to time. Movement will not be strictly one directional. On any given day, a person may feel more anxious or depressed than usual. This occurrence would be represented by slight movement to the left on the continuum. It is tempting to suggest that it is times like these when exercise could prove most beneficial. The evidence present in *Foundations of Exercise and Mental Health* will establish that exercise is associated with both short-term and long-term improvements in the participant. Involvement in a chronic exercise program, therefore, has the potential both to treat and prevent psychological problems. This relationship has been depicted in Figure 1.1.

Exercise and Mental Health: Suggested Mechanisms of Change

Several hypotheses have been advanced as possible mechanisms to explain improved mental health following involvement in a chronic exercise program. This section will provide a brief overview of the endorphin, monoamine, thermogenic, and distraction hypotheses. In addition, an opponent-process model, as well as several other psychological explanations, will be introduced. In the following chapters, each of these hypotheses will be further explored as it relates to specific psychological constructs.

The Endorphin Hypothesis

Despite the absence of compelling scientific evidence, the endorphin hypothesis represents the most popular explanation of the psychological benefits of exercise. When endorphins were discovered (J. Hughes et al.,1975), they were termed the brain's own morphine because of their ability to ease pain, and in some cases, produce a feeling of euphoria. The term endorphin is a general classification label for beta-endorphins, met-enkephalins, and leu-enkephalins. Each of these important body chemicals is a peptide and mimics the chemical structure of morphine. They are particularly important in regulating emotion and perceiving pain.

Early animal research on the brain tissue of rats revealed significant increases in opiate-receptor-site occupancy after they had been forced to run in an activity wheel or swim in cold water (Pert & Bowie, 1979; Wardlaw & Frantz, 1980). It has also been demonstrated by Christie and Chesher (1982) that mice will become "swimming junkies" if they work out regularly. They exhibit the same dependency as that produced by morphine, demonstrating typical withdrawal symptoms when injected with naloxone, an antagonist drug that interferes with beta-endorphin locking into opiate receptor sites. Although science is routinely able to measure this brain activity in rats, we obviously cannot examine beta-endorphin receptor-site occupancy in humans.

Research on the effects of exercise on beta-endorphin levels in humans has necessarily been restricted to measuring levels of beta-endorphin and its metabolites in our peripheral blood (the blood outside the blood-brain barrier). Acknowledging the fact that such measures do not accurately reflect what is actually happening in our brains, research has attempted to examine beta-endorphin levels in our peripheral blood after exercise (Durden-Smith, 1978; Riggs, 1981; Sachs, 1984a; Snyder, 1977a, 1977b, 1980; Villet, 1978). These studies, taken cumulatively, suggest a positive relationship between exercise and psychological well-being and infer the relationship is linked to beta-endorphin levels.

Research has shown that endorphins are released from the pituitary during stress in approximately the same quantities as the stress-related adrenocorticotropic hormone (Rossier, Bloom, & Guillemin, 1980). It is, therefore, not surprising to find that exercise, which causes stress on the body, actually lowers sensitivity to pain. A study by Haier, Quaid, and Mills (1981) revealed that 15 subjects who ran one mile could all withstand the pain of a three-pound weight on the tips of their index fingers almost 70% longer than they could before the run. When the subjects were asked to repeat the run after receiving a shot of naloxone (a drug that suppresses endorphin activity in the brain), the subjects lost their protection against pain. This finding strongly suggests the endorphins caused the increased pain tolerance.

Appenzeller, Standefer, Appenzeller, & Atkinson (1980) sum up the collective research as follows:

Endurance running produces a marked increase in beta-endorphin. Whether this increase persists after physical activity and is responsible for the runner's high, the behavioral alterations of endurance-trained individual's improved libido, heightened pain threshold, absence of depression, and other anecdotal effects of endurance training remains conjectural. (p. 419)

This quote raises several important questions. For example, if endorphins are responsible, why don't all exercisers/runners experience the "runner's high"? Does the endorphins mechanism somehow work differently for these individuals? Why do the behavioral alterations mentioned above remain conjectural? These questions highlight the importance of the integrated approach to research in this area. As previously mentioned, research on the endorphins has been primarily concerned with endorphins taken from the bloodstream. These peripheral measurements require us to question the effects of exercise on endorphins at the central level. Recent work by Farrell (1989), for example, has demonstrated that exercise does not alter the blood-brain barrier in a manner that allows peripheral endorphins to act directly upon the brain. Farrell's findings support the notion that endorphin action is limited to the periphery (e.g., heart). Until it can be shown unequivocally that exercise alters the blood-brain barrier, central effects remain at best speculative. These and similar concerns have led Morgan (1985) to conclude that the endorphin hypothesis can be accepted or rejected solely on the basis of the research studies one chooses to accept or reject. Steinberg and Sykes (1985) agree, stating that the exercise, elevated endorphin, and improved mood relationship is neither straightforward nor conclusive.

Clearly, there is much left to be resolved in this area. On the basis of this and similar reviews (Biddle & Fox, 1989; D.R. Brown, 1990; Hamachek, 1987; Morgan, 1985; Panksepp, 1986; Sachs, 1984b; Sforzo, 1988; Sime, 1990; Steinberg & Sykes, 1985; Thoren, Floras, Hoffman, & Seals, 1990), there appears reason for guarded optimism that future studies will reveal exercise-induced endorphins play a significant role in promoting psychological well-being.

The Monoamine Hypothesis

The monoamine hypothesis suggests the improved affect associated with exercise can be explained by changes in one or more of the brain monoamines (i.e., dopamine, norepinephrine, and serotonin). Until recently, the relationship between our behavior and brain neurochemistry had remained a mystery. Our brain was considered an inaccessible "black box." Although the brain still remains somewhat of a mystery, space-age technology has now allowed neurochemists to commence exploring the biological aspects of psychology. It has now been established that certain areas of the brain and particular neural pathways form systems that are associated with mental processes such as anxiety, depression, pleasure, pain, and even organized thought. Each system utilizes particular neurotransmitters (chemical messengers) that transmit signals across synapses (gaps) between neurons making up the system. Messages travel along the neural pathways in the form of electrical energy. When this electrical energy terminates at the end of a presynaptic neuron, it releases neurotransmitters. These neurotransmitters travel across the synaptic gap and bind onto specific receptor sites (much as a specific key fits a specific lock). If enough neurotransmitters bind onto receptor sites, the message is transmitted. If a sufficient number of neurotransmitters are not present, the message is not transmitted. Of special interest to this publication is the finding that the number of these neurotransmitters available at synapses along particular neural pathways has been related to our moods, which in turn are affected by such things as drugs and exercise. Because an association exists between exercise and improved affect, research has investigated the relationship between physical activity and the monoamines.

Animal research has shown that "rat athletes" have significantly higher levels of both norepinephrine and serotonin in their brains following running or swimming workouts (Barchas & Freedman, 1962; B.S. Brown, Payne, Kin, Moore, & Martin, 1979; B.S. Brown & Van Huss, 1973). Additional studies have shown that rats suffering from stress-induced depression have lower norepinephrine levels in their brains (J.M. Weiss, 1982). It has also been shown that regular running and swimming reduce emotionality in rats (Tharp & Carson, 1975; Weber & Lee, 1968).

Research on the effects of exercise on monoamine activity in humans has been restricted mostly to assessing levels of the urinary metabolite of epinephrine, namely 3-methoxy-4-hydroxyphenolglycol (MHPG). Because brain norepinephrine is unable to cross the blood-brain barrier, research has been restricted to these metabolites of norepinephrine found in cerebrospinal fluid, blood, or urine. Although cerebrospinal fluid measures provide the most direct indication of brain levels of norepinephrine, blood and urine samples are safer and easier to obtain. Because the technology required to detect MHPG in blood plasma is relatively recent, most research has utilized the urinary source of MHPG.

Research has now revealed that regular exercise alters both plasma and urinary levels of MHPG (Doctor & Sharkey, 1971; D. Pierce, Kupprat, &

Harry, 1976). In fact, blood plasma and urinary levels of MHPG have been shown to increase 200% to 600% the normal levels during bouts of acute exercise (Howley, 1981). A study on endurance athletes reports that experienced runners competing in a marathon experience norepinephrine and dopamine plasma levels that are 300% above normal (Appenzeller & Schade, 1979). This elevated level is maintained until the 26-mile race ends, then peaks to 600% normal levels before dropping back to normal levels in about one hour. A study examining the effect of short-term bicycle work at mild, moderate, and heavy workloads suggests that exercise intensity may be an important variable (Hartley et al., 1972). In this study, mild exercise was found to have little effect on plasma MHPG, but moderate and heavy workouts resulted in significant elevations.

Plasma dopamine concentrations are also reportedly affected by exercise (Van Loon, Schwartz, & Sole, 1979). These researchers report significant elevations in plasma dopamine at heart rates of 150% of resting, as well as maximal heart rates. As indicated by Riggs (1981), however, the functional significance of this rise in dopamine is unknown.

As in the case of endorphins, we still do not know what happens to monoamine levels in human brains. Although research measurements remain by necessity indirect, the hypothesis that exercise impacts on mental health by means of monoamine activity is a compelling one. On the basis of the present and similar reviews (Biddle & Fox, 1989; D.R. Brown, 1990; Dienstbier, 1989; Johnsgard, 1989; Morgan, 1988; Riggs, 1981; Sime, 1990), there is ample reason to speculate a monoamine relationship between exercise and mental health. Future studies will undoubtedly contribute to a more thorough understanding of such a relationship.

The Thermogenic Hypothesis

A somewhat different view of the exercise and mental health relationship is termed the thermogenic hypothesis. This idea is by no means a new one. The therapeutic effect of elevating body temperature has been used for many centuries. The practice has been traced back to at least 800 A.D. in Finland (Morgan, 1988). Scandinavians partake in regular sauna baths for both health benefits and the sensation of well-being. This practice appears to possess a fair degree of merit, because research has shown that whole body warming (e.g., warm shower, sauna bathing, or fever therapy) has been shown to reduce muscle tension (deVries, Beckman, Huber, & Dieckmeir, 1968).

It is interesting to speculate how elevated body temperatures are related to improved mental health. Cannon and Kluger (1983) have pointed out that our bodies respond to strenuous exercise in the same manner as when they are invaded by bacteria or viruses. The release of pyrogens (endogenous leucocyte mediators) results in reductions of zinc and iron concentrations in our blood, an increase in leucocytes (white blood cells), and an increase in body temperature (a fever). This combined effect serves to kill off the bacteria and/or virus. It also results in a relaxation effect, just like a sauna or hot shower.

Research by Horne and Staff (1983) provides additional support for the thermogenic hypothesis. Eight trained subjects were exposed to the following three conditions: (a) two 40-minute treadmill runs at 80% VO2 max., separated by a 30-minute rest period; (b) two 80-minute treadmill runs at 40% VO2 max., separated by a 15-minute rest period; and (c) two 40-minute sessions sitting in a hot bath, separated by a 30-minute rest period. The last experimental condition utilized a water temperature that resulted in the same core rectal temperatures in the subjects as was produced with the high intensity exercise treatment. Horne and Staff concluded that high intensity exercise and passive heating produce similar increases in slow wave sleep, and that:

a high and sustained rate of body heating for 1 to 2 hours, particularly the inherent rapid rates of core temperature increase and of body dehydration, may trigger a slow wave sleep response, and that exercise may simply be a vehicle for these effects. (p. 36)

Because slow wave sleep is that portion of the sleep cycle most conducive to relaxation and renewal effects, exercise may indeed have potential to result in mental health benefits.

On a more practical dimension, Johnsgard (1989) has suggested that the pyrogenic response may explain why regular exercisers (who do not overdo it) report fewer incidences and less severity of the common cold or the flu. The pyrogenic effect of exercise, by increasing leucocytes, may kill off the bacteria and viruses associated with these nagging illnesses. If true, this would indeed be an added benefit to the hypothesized thermogenic- produced mental health benefits associated with exercise.

In summary, the research cited above suggests the thermogenic hypothesis is a tenable explanation of the exercise and mental health relationship. However, as Morgan (1988) in his excellent review of this topic suggests, the confirmation or refutation of the thermogenic hypothesis awaits future research.

The Distraction Hypothesis

In contrast to the previous three explanations, which use physiological mechanisms to explain the exercise and mental health relationship, Bahrke and Morgan's (1978) distraction hypothesis proposes a psychological mechanism. This explanation maintains that being distracted from stressful stimuli, or taking "time out" from daily routine activities, is responsible for the improvements in mental health associated with exercise. As Morgan (1988) and Morgan and O'Connor (1989) have stated, this hypothesis does not dispute the influence of physiological mechanisms. It is possible, however, that the psychological effects often attributed to exercise may actually be caused by factors that covary with exercise.

It is important for future research to compare the effects of exercise distraction with other forms of distraction, such as reading, watching TV, resting quietly, meditating, or using a variety of relaxation techniques. An experiment of this nature would allow us to determine if it is the exercise per se, or merely the distraction, which results in positive psychological benefits. On the basis of the aforementioned endorphin, monoamine, and thermogenic hypotheses, it seems reasonable to expect that exercise would be associated with the greatest mental health benefits. Research of this nature, with replicative experiments, is needed to determine the relative value of exercise versus distraction in promoting mental health.

The Opponent-Process Model

Another conceptual explanation for the exercise and mental health relationship is the opponent-process theory of acquired motivation (R.L. Solomon, 1980; R.L. Solomon & Corbit, 1973, 1974). This model is somewhat unique in that it utilizes a physiological mechanism (e.g., endorphins) to explain a physiological change. The basic assumption of this model is that the brain is organized to oppose pleasurable or aversive emotional processes. The body is believed to accomplish this by producing an "opponent" reaction to counter an arousing stimulus. According to R.L. Solomon (1980), stimulus onset produces an increase in sympathetic nervous system activity, and this is termed the *a process*. The *a process* then arouses the opponent, or *b process* in an attempt to restore the organism to homeostasis. The major implication of this model is that with long term exposure to a stimulus (e.g., exercise), the *a process* (e.g., the negative affect associated with exercise) remains constant while the opponent-process (e.g., relaxation) becomes increasingly stronger. This shift in the *b process* may, therefore, be responsible for the positive mental benefits of exercise. The reader seeking additional information on this model is referred to Petruzzello, Landers, Hatfield, Kubitz, and Salazar (1991).

Other Possible Psychological Explanations

Several additional psychological variables have also been suggested in terms of their potential to explain the exercise and mental health relationship. Self-efficacy, or the strength of belief that one can successfully execute a behavior, is one such viewpoint. Bandura (1977) popularized this theory and suggests that a person's perception of his or her ability to perform in demanding situations (e.g., exercise) affects that person's emotions. Self-efficacy can be improved by past performance accomplishments, vicarious experience, verbal persuasion, or level of arousal. The basic tenet of this theory maintains that as a person engages in exercise and experiences fitness gains or bodily changes, self-efficacy improves. This results in the person's feeling better about him or herself and may partially explain the positive benefits of exercise on mental health. Other researchers have termed this process self-mastery (Ismail & Trachtman, 1973), perceived self-confidence (Harter, 1978), and self-esteem (Sonstroem, 1984). Each of these positions will be examined in more detail as it relates to specific psychological constructs.

A final possible explanation of the exercise and mental health relationship has its roots in field theory (Festinger, 1957). Festinger's theory would suggest that people report feeling better after exercise due to cognitive dissonance. Cognitive dissonance occurs whenever a person holds incompatible cognitions. Petruzzello et al. (1991) suggest that people who continue to exercise must find a way to justify their exercise behavior, thereby overcoming the initial negative affect associated with exercise. Cognitive dissonance theory would, therefore, predict that the person's attitude, as well as mood, would shift in a more positive direction. This occurrence may, therefore, be responsible for positive mental changes following participation in chroninc exercise. The authors hasten to point out, however, that no empirical support has yet been established to support the cognitive dissonance hypothesis.

The Exercise and Mental Health Hypotheses: Possible Interaction Effects

Four independent exercise and mental health hypotheses have been advanced. Although these hypotheses were discussed independently, the possibility exists that they may operate in an interactive fashion. Morgan (1988), for example, states that temperature elevations may influence the release, synthesis, or uptake of certain brain monoamines. This would suggest that changes in brain monoamines after exercise may be due to increased brain temperature rather than exercise itself. A more plausible explanation is that the two hypotheses (monoamine and thermogenic) interact in a synergistic fashion. No research has yet attempted to isolate this possible interactive effect.

Another interactive argument is provided by Hamachek (1987), who suggests a possible interaction between endorphins and monoamines. When an individual participates in an aerobic activity for 15 minutes or longer, the body is put into a stress condition. Selye (1974) has defined this state as the body's nonspecific response to any demand placed on it, and the trigger for a chain reaction of physiological changes. One physiological change already discussed is an increase in catecholamines, which seem to exert their greatest effect on the sympathetic nervous system. This results in increased blood pressure, heart rate, metabolism, and other physical reactions that prepare the body for action -- "the fight or flight response." Endorphins, on the other hand, appear to be more related to the parasympathetic system. The aforementioned action serves to lower blood pressure, slow down the heart rate and metabolism, and calm excessive motor activity (Bolles & Fanselow, 1982). Hamachek (1987) has postulated that since both endorphin and catecholamine (monoamine) levels are elevated during exercise, the result may be to increase one's stress-tolerance level. Because the functions of the endorphins and monoamines are antagonistic, stimulation of both systems by exercise possibly results in a physiological striving for equilibrium. The strengthening and balancing of both systems is believed to result in increased stress-tolerance. This viewpoint suggests an interactive effect of the monoamine and endorphin hypotheses.

Finally, the distraction hypothesis probably interacts with, or supplements, each of the other three exercise and mental health hypotheses. Everyone can, at sometime or another, use some "time out" from daily stressors. It seems reasonable to assume an interactive or additive relationship exists among the four hypotheses. When viewed in this light, it is easy to accept the possibility of positive mental health benefits resulting from exercise. Research is still needed to isolate more clearly the exact relationship among the exercise and mental health hypotheses.

The major concern of this book is to examine the relationship between exercise and mental health. Let us, therefore, turn our attention to the empirical research that has focused on specific mental health benefits associated with exercise.

Summary and Conclusions

Modern society appears to be characterized by a relatively high incidence of mental disorders. For some individuals, these problems are severe enough to be considered clinical in magnitude. Problems of this nature invariably require professional intervention. For others, these fluctuations in mental states simply reflect normal reactions to day-to-day stressors. Accumulating research now suggests exercise has the potential to help both types of individuals. Traditionally, the role of exercise as a health behavior focused almost exclusively on physiological adaptations to physical activity. The current trend towards holistic health/wellness has now resulted in exercises being considered for their possible impact on psychological as well as physiological health. In attempting to explain the exercise and mental health relationship, endorphin, monoamine, thermogenic, and distraction hypotheses have been developed. In addition, an opponent-process model as well as several psychological explanations was advanced. At present, no one hypothesis appears superior to the others in explaining how exercise may impact on mental health.

Suggested Readings

Biddle, S.J., & Fox, K.R. (1989). Exercise and health psychology: Emerging relationships. *British Journal of Medical Psychology, 62*, 205-216.

Cannon, J.G., & Kluger, M.J. (1983). Endogenous pyrogen activity in human plasma after exercise. *Science, 220*, 617-619.

Dishman, R.K. (1986). Mental health. In V. Seefeldt (Ed.) *Physical activity and well-being* (pp. 304-340). Reston, VA: American Association for Health, Physical Education, and Recreation Publications.

Morgan, W.P. (1988). Exercise and mental health. In R.K. Dishman Ed.), *Exercise adherence: Its impact on public health* (pp. 91-121). Champaign, IL: Human Kinetics.

Morgan, W.P., & O'Connor, P.J. (1989). Psychological effects of exercise and sports. In E. Ryan, & R. Allman (Eds.), *Sports Medicine,* (pp. 671-689). New York: Academic Press.

Raglin, J.S. (1990). Exercise and mental health: Beneficial and detrimental effects. *Sports medicine, 9,* 323-329.

Regier, D.A., Boyd, J.H., Burke, J.D., Rae, D.S., & Myers, J.K. (1988). One-month prevalence of mental disorders in the United States. *Archives of General Psychiatry, 45,* 977-986.

Sime, W.E. (1990). Discussion: Exercise, fitness, and mental health. In R. Bouchard, R. Shephard, T. Stephens, J. Sutton, & B. McPherson (Eds.), *Exercise, fitness, and health* (pp. 627-633). Champaign, IL: Human Kinetics.

Chapter 2

EXERCISE AND DEPRESSION

As an emotional state, depression is experienced by most of us at some-time in our lives as we deal with frustrations and stress within the context of daily living (Shepel, 1984). It is absolutely normal to experience temporary mood swings. Normal depression is transient and very reactive to situational stressors. Clinical depression, however, is less common and a potentially lethal and debilitating disease. It represents a serious state of psychological malaise and self-dejection. The National Institute of Mental Health study (Regier et al., 1984) portrayed depression as the third most prevalent psychological disorder, afflicting approximately 6% (9.4 million) of the American population.

The objectives of this chapter are to (a) introduce and define clinical and nonclinical depression, (b) review traditional treatments for depression, (c) introduce exercise as an alternative intervention technique, (d) thoroughly analyze and synthesize the empirical research investigating the exercise and depression relationship, (e) provide exercise prescription guidelines that can be gleaned from completed research, and (f) suggest possible explanations for the antidepressant effects of exercise.

Defining Depression

Depression is a term commonly used both in psychiatry and the general population. Because of psychiatry's greater power to label, confine, and define treatment, depression has become much more than a feeling state in the mental health system. The concept and classification of depression have been criticized from both within and without the psychiatric profession. A paper by Goldstein and Anthony (1988) illustrates how the classification of depression has changed throughout the years. These changes are reflected in comparisons of the *Diagnostic and Statistical Manuals of Mental Disorders* (American Psychiatric Association, 1980, 1987). Many of these changes have been in reaction to changes in the theoretical bases of depression. Where it was once considered a neurotic reaction by Freudian theory, it was later considered a biochemical reaction. This change in viewpoint paralleled the continuing advances in neurophysiological research. Most recently, psychosocial theories have once again become popular. An excellent review of the different theories of depression is provided by Akiskal and McKinney (1975). These authors categorize 10 specific models of depression into the following psychological schools of thought: (a) psychoanalytical, (b) behavioral, (c) sociological, (d) existential, and (e) biological. In spite of the diversity arising from these theories, the American Psychiatric Association has attempted to maintain a scientific and atheoretical stance in its definitions that focus on symptoms and severity (i.e., mild, moderate, and severe) of depression.

Recognizing Clinical Depression

According to the latest version, the *Diagnostic and Statistical Manual of Mental Disorders* (American Psychiatric Association, 1987), a Major Depressive Episode is categorized by either a depressed mood or a loss of interest or pleasure in all or most activities, and the presence of other associated symptoms for at least a 2-week period. These symptoms must be persistent and represent a marked change from previous functioning. At least five of the following associated features are also needed: (a) loss of appetite, (b) weight loss or gain, (c) disturbance of sleep, (d) psychomotor agitation or retardation, (e) decrease in energy, (f) sense of worthlessness, (g) guilt, (h) difficulty in concentration, and (i) thoughts of suicide. It is noted that depression may be reactive (precipitated by life events) or endogenous (precipitated by internal, unknown events). In either case, treatment is often prescribed.

Recognizing Nonclinical Depression

Problems with depression are by no means restricted to individuals from the psychiatric population. Generalized, nonclinical depression is experienced by almost everyone over the course of a lifetime. Normal depression is usually tied to some type of identifiable environmental stressor. Grief or loss represent the most common causes of nonclinical depression. The loss may be job related (e.g., termination, transfer, failure to get promoted, or retirement) or involve a form of separation (e.g., death of a pet, a failed romance, divorce, or leaving home). People also commonly experience depression when they finish an important project. Reaching an important goal often feels anticlimactic, with the outcome failing to justify the investment of time and effort, and anticipation. These periods of depression are quite normal and are hence referred to as nonclinical depression. It is only when our depressive episodes go beyond the normal boundaries in terms of frequency, intensity, and duration that we suffer from a mood disorder that could be labeled clinical depression.

Traditional Treatments for Depression

Nonclinical depressive episodes almost always subside in a short period of time without intervention. Similarily, some instances of mild to moderate clinical depression experience spontaneous remission within 6 months of onset. Many individuals have, however, turned to professional help for dealing with their symptoms of depression.

One of the earliest treatments for depression involved the use of psychotherapy. Johnsgard (1989) sums up the efficacy of psychotherapy as follows: "An analysis of hundreds of studies concerning the outcome of psychotherapy suggests it is moderately helpful and somewhat better than no treatment" (p. 116). He further points out that all forms of psychotherapy appear equally effective. Dishman (1986) has suggested that although psychotherapy is often effective with mild and moderate depression, it is often supplemented with antidepressive medications. Severe depression almost always requires medication.

The most widely prescribed antidepressant drugs are the tricyclic antidepressants (TADs). Common TADs include Surmontil, Elavil, and Tofranil. Although these medications are usually effective within about 3 weeks, they are not without a down side. Tricyclic antidepressants typically cause side effects such as blurred vision, dry mouth, and orthostatic hypotension (J.W. Long, 1991; Sternl, Chilnick, Simon & Silverman, 1990). If patients fail to respond to the tricyclic antidepressants, they are often prescribed monoamine oxidase inhibitors (MAOIs). Common MAOIs include Nardil, Parnate, and Marplan. Although the MAOIs do relieve depression, they are also often accompanied by dangerous and potentially lethal side effects. The more critical side effects associated with the MAOIs include dangerous interactions with many foods and drugs, conduciveness to hypertensive crises, and disordered heart rate and rhythm (J.W. Long, 1991; Stern et al., 1990). Because of the serious nature of these potential reactions, the MAOIs are prescribed only if the tricyclic antidepressants do not work.

The treatment of one final category of depression warrants mention. The preceding treatments have all focused on unipolar (mood downswing only) depression. Another illness referred to as bipolar affective disorder (previously called manic-depression) exhibits symptoms of mood downswing (depression) and/or mood upswing (mania). Treatment for bipolar affective disorder almost invariably involves lithium medication. To date, nothing else has worked better (Fieve, 1989; Snyder, 1980). As with other drugs, lithium also has some side effects. It can cause lethargy, affect muscular coordination, and cause fine hand tremor. Long- term use has occasionally been associated with kidney malfunction (Johnsgard, 1989; J.W. Long, 1991; Stern et al., 1990).

In summary, the efficacy of the psychotherapies as well as the negative side effects associated with the chemotherapies highlights the need for a more positive treatment alternative. An accumulating body of research suggests that exercise may have the potential to fill this role.

The Exercise and Depression Relationship

The first empirical study investigating the effect of exercise on depression was performed by Franz and Hamilton (1905), who found a "retarding" effect of exercise on depression. Although this study was a pioneer effort, it appeared to have limited impact on future research. The study was seldom cited and served a minimal heuristic function. The early literature reviews on exercise and mental health (Cureton, 1963; Layman, 1960, 1972; Morgan, 1969) focused mainly upon general mental and/or emotional health rather than specific psychological constructs. During the past two decades, however, this focus appears to have changed. A substantial body of research has accumulated suggesting that exercise is associated with reductions in psychometrically assessed symptoms of depression. The psychometric instruments most frequently employed include the Beck Depression Inventory (Beck, Ward, Mendelson, Mock, & Erbaugh, 1961), the Zung Self-Rating Depression Scale (Zung, 1965), and the Profile of Mood States (McNair, Lorr, & Droppleman, 1971). The MMPI depression scale (Hathaway &

McKinley, 1943), which has been praised as the best discriminator between fit and unfit individuals (Lobstein, Mosbacher, & Ismail, 1983), has also been employed as a testing instrument.

Types of Exercise Associated With Reductions in Depression

Significant reductions in depression have been reported following participation in exercises such as running (Bosscher, 1993; Brown, Ramivez, & Taub, 1978; Doyne et al., 1987; Federici, 1986; Fremont & Craighead, 1987; Greist et al., 1979; Kavanaugh, Shephard, Tuck, & Qureshi, 1977; King, Barr Taylor, & Haskell, 1993; Labbe, Welsh, & Delaney, 1988; Martinsen, 1990; McCann & Holmes, 1984; Palmer, 1985; D.L. Roth & Holmes, 1987; C.B. Taylor, Houston-Miller, Ahn, Haskell, & DeBusk, 1986), walking (Doyne et al., 1987; Emery & Gatz, 1990; Greist et al., 1979; Labbe et al., 1988; Martinsen, Hoffart, & Solberg, 1989b; D.L. Roth & Holmes, 1987), aerobic dance (Jewell, 1987; McCann & Holmes, 1984; Pappas, Golin, & Meyer, 1990), cycling (D.L. Brown, 1984; Doyne, Chambless, & Beutler, 1983; Pelham & Campagna, 1991), weight training (Doyne et al., 1987), karate (Madden, 1990), racquetball (Pappas et al., 1990), jumping rope (Taxe, 1985), and several unspecified aerobic activities (Emery, 1986; Martinsen & Medhus, 1989; Martinsen, Medhus, & Sandvik, 1985; Steege & Blumenthal, 1993). No change in depression has also been reported following participation in running (De Geus, Lorenz, Van Doornen, & Orlebeke, 1993; Eby, 1985; Hannaford, Harrell, & Cox, 1988; King, Barr Taylor, Haskell, & DeBusk, 1989), walking (T.W. Pierce, Madden, Siegel, & Blumenthal, 1993; Sexton, Maere, & Dahl, 1989), and an unspecified aerobic program (Frederick & Ryan, 1993; Martinsen & Medhus, 1989).

> **Prescription Guideline 2.1**
> Running and walking are the two types of physical activity most often associated with significant reductions in participant depression. The majority of studies utilizing these exercise modes report beneficial effects.

Because other physical activities have also been associated with decreases in participant depression, it becomes important to determine if certain types of exercise are more effective than others in terms of producing benefical results.

Comparing exercise types. Only a small number of research studies have attempted to compare different exercise types in terms of their potential to decrease depression in the participants. Eby (1985), utilizing male and female college students, compared running, weight lifting, and running plus weight lifting in terms of their ability to impact on depression. The results of this study indicated that none of the exercise groups experienced reductions in depression and that no differences appeared to exist between groups. A similar study by Doyne et al. (1987) randomly assigned 40 adult females to aerobic (running), anaerobic (weight lifting), or waiting-list control groups. In this study, both exercise groups resulted in significant decreases in depression. An important corollary of this study was that no differences existed between the aerobic and anaerobic exercise groups in terms of their depression-reducing effects. Martinsen et al. (1989b) report similar findings with a sample of 99 male and female clinically depressed adults. In this experiment, subjects were randomly assigned to either an aerobic (walk/jog) or anaerobic (strength & flexibility training) exercise group. After an 8-week training program, both groups experienced significant improvements in depression as measured by the Montgomery and Asberg Depression Rating Scale (Montgomery & Asberg, 1979). Once again, no significant differences were found between the aerobic and anaerobic exercise conditions. The results of this study are provided in Figure 2.1.

Finally, Pappas et al. (1990) compared aerobic dance with aerobic racquetball over a 10-week period with 51 female adults. Significant reductions in depression were experienced in each group, while no significant differences were found between groups. Both types of aerobic exercise were associated with decreased depression.

Prescription Guideline 2.2
   Research has not yet identified one particular type of exercise as being superior in terms of its potential to reduce depression in the participant. Both aerobic and anaerobic exercise sessions appear equally effective.

Future research should attempt to compare different types of aerobic exercise by randomly assigning subjects to groups and groups to treatments. A similar line of research should be performed to compare different types of anaerobic exercises. Finally, various aerobic exercises should be compared with various anaerobic exercises to determine the relative value of the two

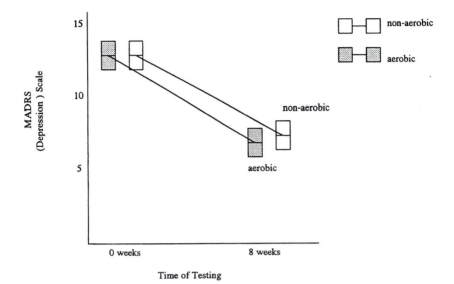

Figure 2.1. Mean score of the Montgomery and Asberg Depression Rating Scale (MADRS), with 95% confidence intervals, comparing the effects of aerobic and nonaerobic exercise on participant depression.
Note. From "Comparing aerobic with nonaerobic forms of execrcise in the treatment of clinical depression: A randomized trial" by E.W. Martinsen, A Hoffart, & O. Solberg, 1989, *Comprehensive Psychiatry, 30*, p.328. Copyright © 1989 by W.B. Saunders. Reprinted by permission.

types of exercise. The few studies that have been completed to date suggest that this future research will determine any form of exercise (aerobic or anaerobic) to be effective in reducing depression in the participant.

Length of exercise program. The relationship between length of exercise program and the effect of exercise on depression level has rarely been discussed in the previous literature reviews. A.D. Simons, Epstein, McGowan, Kupfer, and Robertson (1985) did discuss the length of exercise programs in terms of the time required to document a change in cardiovascular conditioning, but not in terms of the optimal program length to decrease depression. Similarly, not a single experimental study was found that attempted to compare different exercise program lengths with reductions in depression in the participants. For this reason, it becomes necessary to turn to completed research in an attempt to determine optimal program length. Training programs have ranged in length from 3 weeks (Taxe, 1985) to 4 years (Kavanaugh et al., 1977). The majority of studies utilized training programs of 10 weeks or longer. Research also exists, however, that demonstrates significant reductions in depression following exercise programs of 9 weeks (Martinsen et al., 1985), 8 weeks (Bosscher, 1993; Doyne et al., 1987; Martinsen et al., 1989b), 6 weeks (D.L. Brown, 1984; Labbe et al., 1988), 4 weeks (Federici, 1986) and 3 weeks (Taxe, 1985).

> **Prescription Guideline 2.3**
> The majority of studies documenting improvements in depression have involved exercise programs of 10-weeks or longer. Although some research has been reported involving improvements with shorter programs, more consistent results can be expected with longer involvement.

It is important for future studies to systematically compare exercise programs of different lengths in terms of their depression-reducing effects. A worthwhile experiment would be to take a particular exercise, such as running or walking, then randomly assign subjects to groups, then groups to treatments of different program lengths (e.g., 4 weeks, 6 weeks, 8 weeks, etc). A one-way ANOVA with post hoc comparisons could then determine the most appropriate length of exercise program for reducing subject depression. It is this author's opinion that these future studies will find even short-term exercise programs to be effective in lowering depression in the participant.

Exercise frequency. With very few exceptions, completed research studies have required exercise to be performed three times per week (e.g, Bosscher, 1993; King et al., 1993; Steege & Blumenthal, 1993). Experiments utilizing exercise frequencies of five times per week (D.L. Brown, 1984; King et al., 1989), four times per week (Doyne et al., 1983, 1987; Pelham & Campagna, 1991; Taxe, 1985) and two times per week (Jewell, 1987; Madden, 1990; Pappas et al., 1990) have also been reported. In each of these studies, with the single exception of the King et al.(1989) experiment, significant improvements in depression have been reported at the conclusion of the exercise program.

Prescription Guideline 2.4
   Completed research suggests that exercise performed three times per week is sufficient to significantly lower participant depression. Although isolated studies have successfully employed greater exercise frequencies, there does not appear to be any added advantage with exercise frequencies of greater than three or four times per week. By staying within this recommended range, the risk of overuse injury will be minimized, and the desire to stay in the program will be maintained.

It appears that exercise is associated with significant improvements in depression scores regardless of the exercise frequency. This observation must be tempered by the fact that no single experiment has attempted to compare different exercise frequencies in terms of their depression-reducing effects. Future research should isolate a particular exercise mode, then randomly assign subjects to groups, then groups to treatments, with the treatments representing different exercise frequencies (e.g., 2x, 3x,...7x per week). An experiment of this nature would allow us to determine if there is an optimal number of exercise sessions per week associated with decreased depression scores. Information of this nature is important. Although the results accumulated to date suggest beneficial effects at any frequency, it seems logical to expect that future research will discover a "range" of optimal exercise frequencies. When exercise is performed below this minimum range, the cumulative effects of the physical activity may not be sufficient to be associated with significant improvements in depression. On the other hand, exercise frequencies exceeding the maximum range may fail to lower depression (or may even increase it) because the number of exercise sessions may be viewed as excessive. In cases of this nature, the participant may simply view the exercise as another form of stressor, or something else to worry about fitting into an already busy day. This viewpoint is supported by research conducted on overtraining and staleness (Morgan, Brown, Raglin, O'Connor, & Ellickson, 1987; Morgan, Costill, Flynn, Raglin, & O'Connor, 1988; Raglin, 1990, 1993; Veale, 1991). These investigations suggest there is some sort of threshold that, when exceeded, results in worsened mood state and elevated depression.

   Exercise intensity. Analysis of completed research supports earlier criticisms (Doan & Scherman, 1987; Folkins & Sime, 1981; Leith & Taylor, 1990) that exercise intensity has not been consistently documented in research of this nature. Studies that do report on this important variable have documented significant improvements in depression following exercise intensities of 80% VO2 max. (Ossip-Klein et al., 1989), 75% maximum heart rate (Roth & Holmes, 1987), ≥ 60% maximum heart rate (D.L. Brown, 1984; Doyne et al., 1983, 1987; Emery & Gatz, 1990; Hannaford et al., 1988; Palmer, 1985; Pelham & Campagna, 1991; Sexton et al., 1989), ≥ 60% VO2 max. (Bosscher, 1993; Labbe et al., 1988; Martinsen et al., 1989b; Steege & Blumenthal, 1993), 50%-70% maximum heart rate (Doyne et al., 1987; Taxe, 1985), and 50%-70% VO2 max. (Martinsen, 1990; Martinsen et al., 1985; Ossip-Klein et al., 1989). No changes in depression have also been reported, however, at exercise intensities of 60%-80% maximum heart rate (De Geus et al., 1993; Hannaford et al., 1988; King et al., 1989; Sexton et al., 1989).

> **Prescription Guideline 2.5**
> Although exercise intensity has not been consistently reported in the literature, those studies that have documented this important information suggest that both high- and moderate- intensity exercise impact equally on participant depression. An important implication of this observation is that the participant may be well advised to employ moderate-intensity exercise, because it is equally effective, yet poses less risk of injury and discomfort.

For some reason, very few studies have attempted to ascertain the effect of low-intensity exercise on participant depression. In fact, not a single study was found reporting exercise intensities of under 50% VO2 max. or 50% maximum heart rate. This finding is somewhat surprising, suggesting an implicit assumption that a certain minimum level of exercise intensity is required to produce improvements in depression. Two recent studies provide cause to question this assumption. Martinsen et al. (1989b), for example, found that a variety of low intensity, anaerobic exercises performed three times per week for 8 weeks resulted in reductions in depression comparable to those found in an aerobic exercise group training at high exercise intensity (70% VO2 max.). Further support for low intensity exercise has been provided by Madden (1990). In this particular experiment, 41 male and female college students took part in a karate class that met two times per week (2-hour classes) for 29 weeks. The exercise intensity was considered low, with ample time provided for instruction and demonstration of technique. At the end of the 29-week program, the subjects were found to have experienced significant reductions in depression.

The previous two studies suggest the possibility that even low-intensity exercise may be associated with reduced depression in the participant. Low-intensity exercise may, therefore, be sufficient to induce fitness gains and other physical health benefits, especially in chronically sedentary individuals. Future studies should experimentally manipulate low levels of exercise intensities (e.g., 50%, 45%, 40%, VO2 max or age-adjusted maximum heart rate) of a particular physical activity, as well as initial fitness levels, in an attempt to answer these important research questions. If, as expected, this research determines even low-level exercise intensities to be associated with improved depression, this finding could radically alter current views of exercise. It may not be necessary to sweat or suffer undue fatigue in order to experience positive psychological benefits. This finding would undoubtedly make exercise a more attractive option for dealing with problems of depression. It would also go a long way in improving exercise adherence in the participants.

Duration of exercise. The American College of Sport Medicine (1991) provides the guideline that exercise must be performed for 15-30 minutes to promote increased cardiorespiratory functioning and enhanced body composition. It has further been suggested that this same time frame would also be sufficient to promote positive mental health (D.R. Brown, 1990; Dishman, 1985, 1986; Morgan, 1988). Studies investigating the exercise and depression relationship have reported significant reductions in depression utilizing exercise durations of 2 hours (Madden, 1990), 1 hour (Emery, 1986; Emery & Gatz, 1990; Greist et al., 1979; Jewell, 1987; King et al., 1993; Labbe et al., 1988; Martinsen, 1990; Martinsen et al., 1985, 1989b; McCann & Holmes, 1984; Pappas et al., 1990; Steege & Blumenthal, 1993), 45 minutes (Bosscher, 1993), 30 minutes (Fremont & Craighead, 1987; Ossip-Klein et al., 1989; Palmer, 1985; Pelham & Campagna, 1991; D.L. Roth & Holmes, 1987), and < 20 minutes (D.L. Brown, 1984; Taxe, 1985). No changes in depression have also been reported following exercise sessions of 1 hour (Eby, 1985; Hannaford et al., 1988; Martinsen & Medhus, 1989), 35 minutes (T.W. Pierce et al., 1993) and 30 minutes (Sexton et al., 1989).

Prescription Guideline 2.6
  Exercise durations of 15-30 minutes appear sufficient to produce both physiological improvements and lowered depression in the participant.

It is interesting to note that only two experiments have utilized exercise durations of 20 minutes or less. D.L. Brown (1984) required a sample of 28 males with chronic obstructive pulmonary disease to perform on a cycle ergometer for 15- to 20- minute sessions. At the conclusion of this 6-week exercise program, the subjects reported significant reductions in depression as measured by a series of unnamed psychometric instruments. A similar exercise duration was employed by Taxe (1985), who asked 64 male and female college students to skip rope for 10-20 minutes, four times per week. At the end of the 3-week exercise program, subjects demonstrated significant improvements in depression. These studies, although few in number, suggest that short duration exercise may also be associated with significant reductions in depression. Future studies should manipulate exercise durations in the 0-20 minute time frame (e.g., 5, 10, 15, or 20 minutes) in an attempt to determine the minimum time exercise must be performed to impact on participant depression. The research will probably reveal that there is nothing magical about the 20-minute time frame. Comparable reductions in depression are predicted with exercise durations of 10 and 15 minutes. This hypothesis awaits future experimentation.

Importance of Fitness Gains

The assessment of initial levels of cardiovascular fitness of participants and the documentation of a certain minimal level of improvement for treatment groups have been considered crucial for research of this nature (Doan & Scherman, 1987; Thompson & Marten, 1984). In many cases, the amelioration of depression has paralleled increased fitness in the subjects (Doyne et al., 1983; Emery, 1986; Jewell, 1987; Kavanaugh et al., 1977; King et al., 1993; Labbe et al., 1988; Martinsen, 1990; Martinsen et al., 1985, 1989b; McCann & Holmes, 1984; Mutrie, 1986; Palmer, 1985; Pelham & Campagna, 1991; D.L. Roth & Holmes, 1987; Steege & Blumenthal, 1993; Tenario, 1986). Only seven studies that reported fitness gains did not witness a corresponding reduction in depression (De Geus et al., 1993; Eby, 1985; Hannaford et al., 1988; King et al., 1989; Kugler, Dimsdale, Hartley, & Sherwood, 1990; T.W. Pierce et al., 1993; Sexton et al., 1989).

Prescription Guideline 2.7

A synthesis of related research suggests that improved cardiovascular fitness is not a necessary prerequisite for reduced depression in the participant. Other components of fitness, such as body composition, muscular strength/endurance, and flexibility, have been seldom investigated.

Doyne et al. (1987) randomly assigned subjects to one of three groups. A running group exercised at 80% maximum heartrate four times per week for 8 weeks. A weightlifting group exercised at 50% to 60% maximum heart rate over 10 training stations for 8 weeks. A third group functioned as a waiting list control. Posttest measures revealed no significant fitness differences between aerobic and nonaerobic exercise conditions, but depression scores were significantly reduced in both exercise groups. No significant overall differences in depression were found between the two exercise conditions. It was also noted that these improvements were reasonably maintained through the one-year follow-up. The results of this study are demonstrated in Figure 2.2. The authors believed the most conservative conclusion to be drawn from these data was that it is clearly not necessary for exercise to produce cardiovascular fitness gains in order to produce significant reductions in depression.

Additional support for the preceding viewpoint is provided by the numerous studies that do not measure or experience fitness gains, yet demonstrate significant improvements in depression (Bosscher, 1993; D.L. Brown, 1984; R.S. Brown et al., 1978; Federici, 1986; Fremont & Craighead, 1987; Greist et al., 1979; Hayden & Allen, 1984; Johnson, 1986; Madden, 1990; McGilley, 1987; Pappas et al., 1990; Sanstead, 1984; Setaro, 1986; Stephens, 1988; C.B. Taylor et al., 1986; Valliant & Asu, 1985; Weaver, 1985). These findings are not surprising in view of recent suggestions that the antidepressant effects of exercise take place within the first few weeks of treatment, prior to subjects' experiencing improved cardiovascular fitness (Doyne et al., 1983; McCann & Holmes, 1984; North, McCullagh, & Tran, 1990). North et al. (1990) have interpreted this relationship to indicate that cardiovascular fitness level may mediate a portion of the antidepressant effect of exercise, but some other psychological and/or biochemical factor must also account for the reduction in participant depression. Recent researach has provided an interesting corollary to this observation. It has now been demonstrated that individuals with initial low levels of fitness are also more

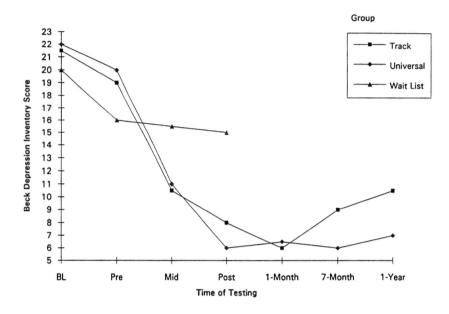

Figure 2.2. Beck Depression Inventory (BDI) scores, comparing the effects of different exercises on participant depression scores.

Note. From "Running versus weight-lifting in the treatment of depression" by E.J. Doyne, D.J. Ossip-Klein, E.D. Bowman, K.M. Osborn, I.B. McDougall-Wilson, & R.A. Neimeyer, 1987, *Journal of Consulting and Clinical Psychology, 55,* p. 752. Copyright © 1987 by the American Psychological Association. Reprinted by permission.

depressed (Berger, 1994; Martinsen, 1993). If this is true, it suggests that sedentary individuals would benefit greatly from participation in an exercise program.

Population Trends

The nature of subjects chosen for experimentation has often been cited as a problem in formulating generalizations from the research findings. It has been suggested that although some research studies involving healthy adults and college students have demonstrated significant reductions in depression, this is not a reliable result among individuals initially scoring within a clinically normal range of depression (D.R. Brown, 1990; Dishman, 1985, 1986; Folkins, Lynch, & Gardner, 1972; Morgan & Pollock, 1978; Morgan,

Roberts, Brand, & Feinerman, 1970; Naughton, Bruhn, & Lategola, 1968; Raglin, 1990; Sime, 1990; J.J. Stern & Cleary, 1982). If this viewpoint is true, it suggests that exercise is more effective as a treatment rather than a preventative measure.

Studies using nonclinical populations. The preceding viewpoint likely originated as a result of a study performed by Morgan et al. (1970). These investigators studied the effect of a 6-week exercise program in a sample of nonclinical adult males. Results of the study indicated that exercise did not result in significant reductions in depression. However, when the authors analyzed a subsample of the individuals who were depressed at the outset of the study, significant reductions were noted. Raglin (1990) interpreted these findings to indicate that exercise does not make normal individuals more normal, but is an effective strategy if the participant is experiencing depression at the time of exercise. Additional support for this position can be gleaned from randomized experimental trials across 20 weeks (Morgan & Pollock, 1978) and 2 years (J.J. Stern & Cleary, 1982), indicating no change from initially normal subject depression scores.

Accumulating research now gives cause to question this original viewpoint. Healthy asymptomatic subjects have been studied in the form of college students (Brown et al., 1978; Federici, 1986; Hayden & Allen, 1984; Jewell, 1987; Johnson, 1986; Madden, 1990; Pappas et al., 1990; D.L. Roth & Holmes, 1987), and adults (De Geus et al., 1993; Frederick & Ryan, 1993; Fremont & Craighead, 1987; King et al., 1989, 1993; Labbe et al., 1988; Setaro, 1986; Steege & Blumenthal, 1993; Stephens, 1988; Weaver, 1985). With only three exceptions (De Geus et al., 1993; Frederick & Ryan, 1993; King et al., 1989), these studies consistently reported significant reductions in depression following their respective exercise programs. In addition, special populations not experiencing clinical problems with depression, including elderly adults (Emery, 1986; Emery & Gatz, 1990; King et al., 1993; Valliant & Asu, 1985), chronic obstructive pulmonary diseased individuals (D.L. Brown, 1984), alcoholics (Palmer, 1985), and postcoronary patients (Kavanaugh et al., 1977; McGilley, 1987; Taylor et al., 1986) have also experienced significant reductions in depression as a result of participation in an exercise program. A recent review by D.R. Brown (1992) however, suggests the results of research with older adults are not so consistent.

The consistency of these research findings certainly highlights the potential for exercise to impact positively on individuals who fall within a normal range of depression. It no longer appears that only clinically depressed individuals can benefit from an exercise program. This observation should come as no surprise. Almost everyone experiences temporary, minor mood swings over the course of a day. Participation in an ongoing exercise program may serve to "buffer" these negative feelings on a day-to-day basis, thereby resulting in lower cumulative depression scores. Regular exercise may, therefore, not only reduce existing depression but also aid in preventing the onset of depression in the participant. Hence, for individuals who are physically active, the primary psychological benefit of exercise may be the maintenance of positive mental health, rather than the treatment of an existing mood state. Support for this position is provided by Stephens (1988), who completed extensive secondary analyses of four large data bases in Canada and the United States over a 10-year period. Stephens concluded "the inescapable conclusion from this study is that the level of physical activity is positively associated with good mental health in the household populations of the United States and Canada" (pp. 41-42). He further reported relatively infrequent symptoms of depression in physically active individuals.

It would be interesting for future studies to compare physically active and physically inactive subjects in terms of day-to-day depression scores, although a study of this nature involves a somewhat different type of construct than do traditional measures of clinical depression. Experiments utilizing single-subject repeated-measures designs would be most appropriate to determine if regular exercisers experience less frequent and intense symptoms of depression. To do this, a measurement instrument that measures both frequency and intensity of depression would be required. Experiments of this nature will portray exercise programs to be associated with less frequent depressive episodes and lower overall depression scores than is the case with nonexercisers. This prediction applies equally to depressed and nondepressed individuals.

Studies using clinical populations. The safety and efficacy of exercise programs in treating clinically depressed patients using medication has been questioned, with early suggestions that exercise could act synergistically to result in patients' overdosing on the antidepressant medication (Kostrabula, 1981). Recent research, however, has demonstrated that exercise does not interact with or potentiate the effects of tricyclic antidepressants (Martinsen, 1987; Martinsen et al., 1985). Hence, exercise has been found to be an effective means of treating clinical depression, and recent evidence suggests it can serve as an adjunct to psychotropic therapy.

Clinically depressed subjects have been researched in the form of college students (McCann & Holmes, 1984) and adults (Bosscher, 1993; Doyne et al., 1983, 1987; Eby, 1985; Greist et al., 1979; Hannaford et al., 1988; Martinsen, 1990; Martinsen et al., 1985, 1989b; Martinsen & Medhus, 1989; Pelham & Campagna, 1991; Sexton et al., 1989). Only four of these studies (Eby, 1985; Hannaford et al., 1988; Martinsen & Medhus, 1989; Sexton et al., 1989) were not associated with significant reductions in depression. It, therefore, appears that exercise is an effective treatment for symptoms of clinical depression.

Several studies have attempted to compare exercise with other more traditional methods of treating clinical depression. Greist et al. (1979) compared the effects of a walk/jog program to two different forms of psychotherapy in a 12-month follow-up of randomly assigned psychiatric outpatients. At the conclusion of the exercise program, it was found that the reduction in depression associated with exercise was equivalent to time-limited psychotherapy and superior to time-unlimited psychotherapy. Furthermore, at the 12-month follow-up, 11 of 12 patients treated with exercise were still asymptomatic, whereas approximately one-half of those individuals receiving the more traditional psychotherapy had returned for treatment. A replication study by M.H. Klein et al. (1985) demonstrated that running therapy and meditation training had similar depression- reducing effects over a 12-week period, with both groups showing superior treatment effects compared with group psychotherapy. The improvements in depression were still apparent at a 9-month follow-up assessment. In a recent replication of his earlier work, Greist (1987) assessed the effects of 12 weeks of exercise, group psychotherapy, or Bensonian relaxation technique in a sample of depressed outpatients. Results of the study indicated that all treatments resulted in similar reductions at the end of the 12-week treatment period. At the 9-month follow-up, however, it was found that the reductions in depression experienced by the exercise and meditation group had persisted, whereas the group therapy treatment displayed some remission. Finally, a recent study by Martinsen and Medhus (1989) assessed 43 patients who had been treated in the hospital for major depression 1 to 2 years after discharge. Subjects were asked to evaluate the different therapeutic modalities they received while at the mental health clinic. These various interventions included medication, community meetings, contact with other patients, group psychotherapy, physical exercise, individual psychotherapy, and contact with the milieu staff. Patients were asked to indicate which intervention they found most helpful and to rank the top three by means of a 3-point scale (with 3 being most helpful). While in hospital, patients had been randomly assigned to a training group and a control group by block randomization with respect to sex. The training group underwent a 6-9 week aerobic training program, while the control group attended occupational therapy. Because six patients in the control group started to exercise at the conclusion of the testing period, they were considered a separate control plus training treatment group. Results of the survey data collected 1-2 years after discharge revealed that patients retrospectively ranked physical exercise as the most important element in their comprehensive treatment program. These findings are demonstrated in Figure 2.3.

The authors interpret these findings to suggest that physical exercise may be a viable alternative treatment for depressed patients who do not respond adequately to the more traditional treatments. They recommend, however, the need for additional replication studies utilizing greater numbers of participants.

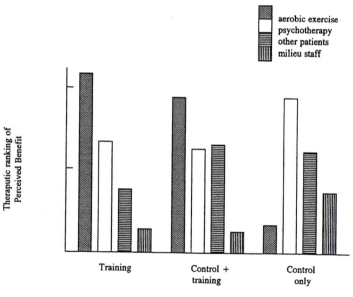

Figure 2.3. Patients' ranking of the most important therapeutic elements in their treatment for depression.
Note. From "Adherence to exercise and patient's evaluation of physical exercise in a comprehensive treatment for depression" by E.W. Martinsen and A. Medhus, 1989, Nordisk-Psykiatrisk-Tidsskrift, 43, p. 413. Copyright © 1990 by the American Psychological Association. Reprinted by permission.

Exercise and Depression: A Meta-Analysis Summary

A recent meta-analytic review by North et al., (1990) provides some tentative answers concerning the exercise and depression relationship. To overcome some of the limitations of traditional reviews, Glass (1976) developed a methodology for the statistical review of literature. Glass, McGaw, and Smith (1981) have described meta-analysis as a statistical analysis of the summary results of a large number of empirical studies. It is a quantitative approach to reviewing research that uses a wide variety of statistical techniques for sorting, classifying, and summarizing information from the findings of many experimental studies. It is further believed that a meta-analysis overcomes many of the problems associated with traditional narrative reviews. For a further review of this statistical technique, the reader is referred to Glass et al. (1981).

By means of the meta-analysis technique, North et al. (1990) have concluded that (a) exercise significantly decreased depression, and the antidepressant effects continued through follow-up measures; (b) subject populations experiencing similar decreases in depression included all age groups, both males and females, as well as clinical populations and nonclinical populations ; (c) all modes of exercise, including anaerobic exercise, were effective in decreasing depression; (d) the longer the exercise program, the greater the decreases in depression; and (e) exercise was at least as effective as other traditional treatments for depression.

Although the North et al. (1990) meta-analysis does an excellent job in sorting and quantifying available research results, it must be remembered that this procedure is unable to remedy any methodological weaknesses inherent in the collated individual research studies. Studies of exemplary experimental rigor are grouped with studies of poor experimental rigor. It would be of significant value to perform a meta-analysis on only those studies employing a true experimental design as defined by Campbell and Stanley (1963). A meta-analytic review of this nature would provide more generalizable results because the analyis would be performed only on well-controlled experiments. Unfortunately, a sufficient number of true experimental designs have not been conducted to make a meta-analysis of this nature feasible. As a viable alternative, a mini-analysis will be performed by summarizing the empirical studies in terms of experimental designs and ensuing results. As a reference point for this mini-analysis, the reader is referred to Table 2.1.

TABLE 2.1
Empirical Research Investigating the Exercise/Depression Relationship

Study	Design	Participants	Controls	Fitness Demonstrated?	Psychological Instruments	Outcome
Bosscher (1993)	Quasi-Experimental	Male and female depressed in patients	No	No	Zung Self-Rating Depression Scale	Improved
D.L. Brown (1984)	Quasi-Experimental	Males with chronic obstructive pulmonary disease	Yes	No	Unnamed Instruments	Improved
R.S. Brown, Ramivez, and Taub (1978)	Quasi-Experimental	College students	Yes	No	Zung Self-Rating Depression Scale	Improved
De Geus, Lorenz, Van Doornen, and Orlebeke (1993)	Quasi-Experimental	Male adults	Yes	Yes	Zung Self-Rating Depression Scale	No Change
Doyne, Chambless, and Beutler (1983)	Quasi-Experimental	Female depressed adults	No	Yes	Schedule for Affective Disorders	Improved
Doyne, Ossip-Klein, Bowman, Osborn, McDougall-Wilson, and Neimeyer (1987)	Experimental	Female depressed adults	Yes	Yes	Beck Depression Inventory, Adjective Checklist, Hamilton Rating Scale for Depression	Improved
Eby (1985)	Experimental	Female depressed adults	Yes	Yes	Zung Self-Rating Depression Scale	No Change
Emery (1986)	Experimental	Male and female elderly adults	Yes	Yes	CES Depression Scale	Improved
Federici (1986)	Quasi-Experimental	Male and female college students	Yes	No	Zung Self-Rating Depression Scale, MMPI(Depression Scale)	Improved
Frederick and Ryan (1993)	Pre-Experimental	Male and female adults	No	No	CES Depression Scale	No Change
Fremont and Craighead (1987)	Quasi-Experimental	Male and female adults	No	No	Beck Depression Inventory, Profile of Mood States	Improved
Greist, Klein, Eischens, Faris, Gurman, and Morgan (1979)	Quasi-Experimental	Male and female adult outpatients (depression)	No	No	Symptom Checklist	Improved
Hannaford, Harrell, and Cox (1988)	Experimental	Male adult psychiatric patients (depression)	Yes	Yes	Zung Self-Rating Depression Scale	No Change
Hayden and Allen (1984)	Pre-Experimental	Male and female college students	No	No	Beck Depression Inventory	Improved

TABLE 2.1   (Cont.)

Study	Design	Participants	Controls	Fitness Demonstrated	Psychological Instruments	Outcome
Jewell (1987)	Quasi-Experimental	Female college students	No	Yes	Beck Depression Inventory, Profile of Mood States	Improved
Johnson (1986)	Experimental	Male and female college students	Yes	No	Zung Self-Rating Depression Scale	Improved
Kavanaugh, Shephard, Tuck, and Qureshi (1988)	Quasi-Experimental	Depressed postcoronary males	No	Yes	MMPI (Depression Scale)	Improved
King, Barr Taylor, and Haskell (1993)	Experimental	Male and female older adults	Yes	Yes	Beck Depression Inventory	Improved
King, Barr Taylor, Haskell, and DeBusk (1989)	Quasi-Experimental	Male and female adults	No	Yes	Unnamed Instrument	No Change
Kugler, Dimsdale, Hartley, and Sherwood (1990)	Quasi-Experimental	Male adults with myocardial infarction	No	Yes	MMPI (Depression Scale)	Improved
Labbe, Welsh, and Delaney (1988)	Quasi-Experimental	Female adult volunteers	No	Yes	Beck Depression Inventory	Improved
Madden (1990)	Quasi-Experimental	Male and female college students	No	No	Zung Depression Scale	Improved
Martinsen (1990)	Quasi-Experimental	Male and female psychiatric patients	No	Yes	Beck Depression Inventory	Improved
Martinsen, Hoffart, and Solberg (1989b)	Quasi-Experimental	Male and female depressed inpatients	No	Yes	Beck Depression Inventory	Improved
Martinsen and Medhus (1989)	Experimental	Male and female depressed inpatients	Yes	No	Beck Depression Inventory	No Change
Martinsen, Medhus, and Sandvik (1985)	Experimental	Male and female depressed adults	Yes	Yes	Beck Depression Inventory	Improved
McCann and Holmes (1984)	Experimental	Female depressed college students	Yes	Yes	Beck Depression Inventory	Improved
McGilley (1987)	Quasi-Experimental	Male adult coronary patients	Yes	No	Unnamed Instruments	Improved

TABLE 2.1   (Cont.)

Study	Design	Participants	Controls	Fitness Demonstrated	Psychological Instruments	Outcome
Mutrie (1986)	Experimental	Male and female depressed adults	Yes	Yes	Beck Depression Inventory, Profile of Mood States	Improved
Palmer (1985)	Quasi-Experimental	Male adult alcoholics	Yes	Yes	Self Rating Depression Scale	Improved
Pappas, Golin, and Meyer (1990)	Quasi-Experimental	Male and female depressed adults	Yes	No	Beck Depression Inventory	Improved
Pelham and Campagna (1991)	Quasi-Experimental	Male and female schizophrenics	No	Yes	Beck Depression Inventory, Mental Health Inventory	Improved
T.W. Pierce, Madden, Siegel, and Blumenthal (1993)	Experimental	Male and female hypertensive adults	Yes	Yes	CES Depression Scale	No Change
D.L. Roth and Holmes (1987)	Experimental	Male and female college students	Yes	Yes	Beck Depression Inventory, Hopkins Symptoms Checklist	Improved
Sanstead (1984)	Quasi-Experimental	Male and female depressed adults	No	No	Beck Depression Inventory	Improved
Setaro (1986)	Quasi-Experimental	Male and female adults	Yes	No	MMPI (Depression Scale)	Improved
Sexton, Maere, and Dahl (1989)	Quasi-Experimental	Male and female neurotics	No	Yes	Beck Depression Inventory, Symptoms Checklist	No Change
Steege and Blumenthal (1993)	Quasi-Experimental	Female premenopausal adults	No	Yes	Menstrual Symptoms Questionnaire	Improved
Stephens (1988)	Pre-Experimental	Male and female adults	No	No	CES Depression Scale	Improved
C.B. Taylor, Houston-Miller, Ahn, Haskell, and DeBusk (1986)	Experimental	Male adult myocardial infarction patients	Yes	No	Beck Hopelessness-Helplessness Scale	Improved
Tenario (1986)	Quasi-Experimental	Female adults (subclinically depressed)	Yes	Yes	CES Depression Scale	Improved
Weaver (1985)	Quasi-Experimental	Female adults	Yes	No	Multiple Affect Adjective Checklist	Improved

Quality of Completed Research - Design Considerations

Before moving on to attempt an explanation of the exercise and depression relationship, and the development of exercise prescription guidelines for the practitioner, it is important to consider the quality of research completed to date. Perhaps the best yardstick for evaluating quality of research is provided by Campbell and Stanley (1963) in the classic text *Experimental and Quasi-Experimental Designs for Research*. These authors categorize research as being pre-experimental, quasi-experimental, or true experimental designs. Pre-experimental research represents the weakest category, utilizing one-shot case studies, one group pretest-posttest designs, or static group comparisons. Quasi-experimental research includes time-series designs, designs with equivalent time samples, designs with equivalent material samples, and nonequivalent control group designs. Finally, true experimental designs involve pretest-posttest control group designs, Solomon four-group designs, and posttest-only control group designs. True experimental research provides optimal control of threats to internal and external validity because of random assignment of participants to groups and random assignment of groups to treatments and controls. Quasi-experimental studies, while providing less control-rigor than true experimental designs, also represent an acceptable form of research because of their applicability to a more natural setting than is the case with true experimental designs.

Forty-two empirical studies are summarized in Table 2.1. Perhaps the most glaring observation that can be made of the collated research pertains to the fact that 34 of the 42 studies (81%) reported significant reductions in depression following exercise. This finding is heartening and speaks well of the potential of exercise in the treatment and prevention of depression. Although it has previously been suggested (Doan & Scherman, 1987; Folkins & Sime, 1981; Leith & Taylor, 1990) that as experimental rigor improves, the positive effects of exercise become less obvious, the findings from Table 2.1 do not completely support such a claim. Of the 42 studies summarized, 2 of 3 (67%) pre-experimental, 23 of 26 (89%) quasi-experimental, and 9 of 13 (69%) true experimental studies reported significant improvements in depression following exercise. Although a slight downward trend is noticeable as experimental rigor improves, the smaller number of pre-experimental and true experimental studies completed make it difficult to formulate such a conclusion. Even though this slight downward trend is noticeable, the fact that 69% of the most rigorous experimental designs reported significant improvements in depression reveals a positive effect from exercise even when experimental designs become more controlled. In addition, the value of utilizing quasi-experimental designs is that although they sacrifice some experimental control, they have the added advantage of improved feasibility, relevance, and the absence of demand characteristics (Leith & Taylor, 1990). Only three studies (Frederick & Ryan, 1993; Hayden & Allen, 1984; Stephens, 1988) utilized the relatively weak pre-experimental designs. It would, therefore, appear that the majority of studies examining the exercise and depression relationship represent relatively sound research. It is also heartening to note that a good mix of quasi-experimental and true experimental research has been conducted. The observation that both field and laboratory research report the same beneficial effects of exercise on depression can only strengthen our position that exercise has excellent potential to impact positively on depression in the participant.

The Exercise and Depression Relationship

The fact that exercise has been consistently associated with reductions in participant depression has led researchers to speculate as to underlying mechanisms of this relationship. Several hypotheses have been advanced in an effort to explain how exercise may affect the psychological construct of depression. It is interesting to note that hypotheses attempting to explain the exercise and mental health relationship differ from our traditional concept of hypotheses. In traditional experimental designs, hypotheses are predictions that are formulated before the experiment proper begins. In this case, however, hypotheses have been developed in an attempt to explain results that have earlier been reported. To date, several hypotheses have been advanced in an attempt to explain the exercise and depression relationship.

The Endorphin Hypothesis

Accumulating evidence suggests that exercise elevates blood-plasma endorphin levels. A study by Carr et al., (1981) recruited seven unconditioned females and exposed them to a rigorous and increasingly intense exercise program for 2 months. As a result of exercising for an hour a day, 6 days a week, their plasma endorphin levels rose dramatically from 57% above normal during the first week all the way up to 145% above normal by the end of the eighth week. This research suggests both an acute and chronic response to exercise. Bortz (1982) has suggested that beta-endorphin levels elevate after only a few minutes of exercise. The Carr et al. (1981) study indicates that the effect is also chronic and continues to build over time. Several other studies report elevated plasma endorphin levels as a result of running programs (Appenzeller, 1980, 1981a, 1981b; Appenzeller & Schade, 1979; Appenzeller et al., 1980; Colt, Wardlaw, & Frantz, 1981; Moore, 1982).

In spite of the fact that research consistently reports elevated beta-endorphin levels after exercise, the hypothesis that exercise-produced endorphins result in improved depression remains tenable. Morgan (1985), for example, has pointed out that even if endorphin levels in our brains and in our peripheral systems do not covary, changes in peripheral opiate levels (which reflect adrenal gland activity) could theoretically affect our emotional states. Similarily, Johnsgard (1989) suggests that it has not been satisfactorily demonstrated that endorphins play a central role in depression. They do, however, appear to be related to feelings of well-being and euphoria. This concept will be fully explored in chapter 6.

The Monoamine Hypothesis

Although the endorphin hypothesis remains questionable, certain other neurotransmitters are receiving increased attention. Many theorists now see the catecholamine (norepinephrine and dopamine) and indolamine (serotonin) neurotransmitter systems as central in depression (Garver & Davis, 1979; Greist et al., 1979; Morgan, 1985; Ransford, 1982; J.M. Weiss, 1982).

To date, a variety of studies have been performed examining acute exercise and urinary MHPG with exercise (Beckman, Ebert, Post, & Goodwin, 1979; Ebert, Post, & Goodwin, 1972; Post, Kotin, & Goodwin, 1973). Other researchers, however, report no significant effects of exercise on urinary MHPG (Sweeney, Leckman, Maas, Hattox, & Heninger, 1980; Sweeney, Maas, & Henninger, 1978). An excellent review of this topic by Morgan (1988) suggests that it is difficult to interpret these results because studies have failed to adequately control for exercise intensity and duration. This makes replication impossible.

Several other studies have investigated the acute exercise and urinary MHPG relationship in nonclinical subjects. A significant increase in plasma MHPG (but not urinary MHPG) followed acute exercise in each of these studies (Goode, Dekirmenjian, Meltzer, & Maas, 1973; Howlett & Jenner, 1978; Peyrin & Pequignot, 1983; Tang, Stancer, Takahashi, Shephard, & Warsh, 1981).

To date, no studies have attempted to ascertain the effects of chronic exercise on either urinary or plasma MHPG. The relationship between physical fitness (VO2 max.) and MHPG has, however, been examined (M.S. Sothman & Ismail, 1984, 1985; M.S. Sothman, Ismail, & Chodko-Zajko, 1984). These studies reported nonsignificant differences in early morning and postwork urinary MHPG between groups divided on the basis of physical fitness.

In summary, as was the case with endorphins, we still do not know what happens to monoamine levels in human brains following exercise. Although the evidence is indirect, the hypothesis that exercise ameliorates depression by activating the monoamine system remains compelling. More replicative research is needed to illuminate this relationship.

Other Possible Explanations

Two other exercise and mental health theories include the thermogenic and distraction hypotheses. To date, no research has been found that attempts to explain the exercise and depression relationship in terms of either the thermogenic or the distraction hypotheses. This lack of research is somewhat surprising. Whereas the thermogenic viewpoint focuses primarily upon anxiety (see chapter 3), the distraction hypothesis has intuitive appeal in terms of explaining the effects of exercise on depression. Johnsgard (1989) has reported that endurance athletes claim it is impossible to train long and hard and be depressed. He further suggests that strenuous exercise and depression are poles apart in terms of feeling states. This viewpoint makes a good deal of sense. When the athlete is concentrating on training goals as well as the feelings associated with a workout (e.g., fatigue, breathing, soreness), it probably takes his or her mind off depressing and troubling thoughts. The same argument holds for the casual exerciser, who devotes undivided attention to completing the workout before running out of breath. In either case, exercise serves as a form of distraction from depressing thoughts. Research is needed to investigate the distraction hypothesis in terms of its potential for explaining the positive effects of exercise on depression. A valuable research study would be to compare participants who utilize task-related or distracting thought content with another group of subjects who do not employ this strategy while exercising. Studies of this nature will demonstrate that the former group will experience more reductions in depression than will the latter group. This prediction would be even stronger if the second group reported thinking depressing thoughts. Future research may, therefore, establish that what we think while exercising may be almost as important as the exercise itself.

Closely related to the preceding point, it is surprising that no research has been conducted investigating the effect of recreational sport leagues on participant depression. Recreational sports not only provide the potential for distraction but also include a social dimension that is often lacking from formal exercise programs. These two features, taken together, would suggest that recreational sports have significant potential for ameliorating participant depression.

A final explanation of the exercise and depression relationship involves the concepts of self-efficacy and skills mastery. Zeiss and Munoz (1979) have suggested that for any treatment intervention to reduce depression, the following criteria are necessary: (a) a rationale providing structure that helps patients believe they can control their own behavior, (b) the teaching of significant skills to the patient, (c) an emphasis on independent use of these skills and personal goal attainment, and (d) attribution of improved mood to the patient's personal skills mastery. It is obvious that exercise programs incorporate all of these elements. It may, therefore, be the case that exercise improves depression in the participant by providing that individual with a feeling of self-confidence for having mastered the particular exercise or physical activity skill. Future studies should attempt to measure changes in self-efficacy and perceived skills mastery and to relate these changes to reductions in depression. Future studies will demonstrate that significant improvements in the former will be associated with significant improvements in the latter. To date, no research has attempted to analyze this proposed relationship.

Summary and Conclusions

Participation in a wide variety of exercise programs appears to be associated with significant reductions in participant depression. To date, no one particular type of exercise has proven superior in terms of its depression-reducing effects. Similarly, no differences have been found between aerobic and anaerobic exercises. Both types of exercise have been consistently associated with improvements in subject depression scores. Completed research suggests exercise should be performed at least three times per week for a minimum of 15 to 20 minutes per session. The actual intensity of exercise does not appear to be related to differential improvements in depression. Although the optimal length of an exercise program has not yet been established, recent research suggests better and more consistent results with longer programs. Changes in aerobic fitness do not appear necessary in order to experience reductions in depression, although less fit individuals appear more depressed initially. All sample populations, including both clinical and nonclinical samples, appear to benefit equally from a chronic exercise program. Finally, the exact mechanism explaining the exercise and depression relationship has not been clearly established. The endorphin and monoamine hypotheses have been most frequently cited, although the opponent-process viewpoint, the distraction hypothesis, and the self-efficacy/skills mastery explanations remain viable alternatives.

Suggested Readings

Dishman, R.K. (1994). Biological psychology, exercise, and stress. *Quest, 46*, 28-59.

Doyne, E.J., Ossip-Klein, D.J., Bowman, E.D., Osborn, K.M., McDougall-Wilson, J.B., & Neimeyer, R.A. (1987). Running versus weight lifting in the treatment of depression. *Journal of Consulting and Clinical Psychology, 55*, 748-754.

Dunn, A.L., & Dishman, R.K. (1991). Exercise and the neurobiology of depression. *Exercise and Sport Sciences Reviews, 19*, 41-98.

Greist, J.H. (1987). Exercise intervention with depressed outpatients. In W. Morgan & S. Goldston (Eds.), *Exercise and mental health* (pp. 117-121). Washington, DC: Hemisphere Publishers.

Martinsen, E.W. (1993). Therapeutic implications of exercise for clinically anxious and depressed patients. *International Journal of Sport Psychology, 24*, 185-199.

Martinsen, E.W., Hoffart, A., & Solberg, O. (1989). Comparing aerobic with nonaerobic forms of exercise in the treatment of clinical depression: A randomized trial. *Comprehensive Psychiatry, 30*, 324-331.

North, T.C., McCullagh, P., & Tran, Z.V. (1990). Effects of exercise on depression. *Exercise and Sport Sciences Reviews, 18*, 379-415.

Pappas, G.A., Golin, S., & Meyer, D.L. (1990). Reducing symptoms of depression with exercise. *Psychsomatics, 31*, 112-113.

Chapter 3

EXERCISE
AND ANXIETY

Periodic anxiety is a normal stress emotion as long as it remains moderate in frequency and intensity. It is simply a reaction to everyday hassles, frustrations, aspirations, and interpersonal relationships. For some individuals, however, the anticipation of real or imaginary problems can become so strong or recurrent that they reach clinical magnitude. When this happens, the resulting anxiety interferes with family relationships, work, and personal well-being. Maladaptive behavior often results, and the symptoms become so painful that it often becomes necessary to seek professional help. Problems of this nature are by no means uncommon. The National Institute of Mental Health study (Regier et al., 1984) reported that the anxiety category represents the highest incidence of mental health problems in America. The condition afflicts approximately 8% (13.1 million) of the American population.

The objectives of this chapter are to (a) introduce the concept and components of anxiety, (b) distinguish between clinical and nonclinical anxiety, (c) provide an overview of the traditional treatments for anxiety, (d) examine the psychophysiological correlates of anxiety, (e) suggest exercise as an appropriate anxiolytic intervention technique for both state and trait anxiety, (f) discuss individual differences and psychophysiological reactivity to stress, (g) provide a thorough synthesis of empirical research investigating the exercise and anxiety relationship, (h) provide exercise prescription guidelines for improving anxiety, and (i) suggest possible explanations of how exercise may impact on participant anxiety.

Defining Anxiety

A great amount of early effort was expended to define anxiety, delineate it, measure its characteristics, and devise ways of reducing it (Freud, 1963;

May, 1977; Sarason & Spielberger, 1976a, 1976b, 1979; Spielberger & Sarason, 1975, 1977, 1978). In its simplest form, anxiety may be defined as a subjective feeling of apprehension and heightened physiological arousal. It is closely associated with our concept of fear. The physiological responses common to anxiety include sweating, rapid heartbeat, muscle tension, and stomach cramps. In addition to these physiological responses, anxiety disorders usually express themselves in intense feelings of psychological distress, along with anticipation of future threat. Research in this area usually distinguishes between state and trait measures of anxiety. State anxiety refers to "right now" types of feelings, whereas trait anxiety involves a general predisposition towards anxiety across a variety of situations. State measures are very transient, often changing within a short period of time, whereas trait anxiety is a relatively stable dimension of the individual's personality. Both of these constructs will be thoroughly explored later in this chapter.

Recognizing Clinical Anxiety

In the *Diagnostic and Statistical Manual of Mental Disorders* (American Psychiatric Association, 1987), phobic disorders and anxiety states represent subcategories of anxiety disorders. The essential difference between phobic disorders and anxiety states is that in phobic disorders, the individual's concern or anxiety is directed toward a quite specific person or situation, such as spiders, snakes, dogs, or open spaces. In contrast, anxiety states represent more generalized, less specific aspects of anxiety.

In some individuals, anxiety can occur with little warning, and with no apparent relationship to a particular cause. This most severe anxiety state is called panic disorder and is marked by episodic anxiety reactions and sustained high levels of psychological tension. A central feature of panic disorder is "free-floating" anxiety; that is, anxiety with no apparent source. For other individuals, a lower level of anxiety is experienced in relation to a wider range of events. This condition is classified a general anxiety disorder and is a chronic, less cyclic version of panic disorder. In almost all cases, clinical anxiety requires professional intervention.

Recognizing Nonclinical Anxiety

Problems with anxiety are not, however, restricted to the psychiatric population. Generalized, subclinical anxiety is experienced by most people at some point in their lives. When individuals experience anxiety states frequently and in many different situations, this condition is referred to as *trait anxiety*. Anxiety of this nature is generalized and represents a chronic pattern. A somewhat different reaction, referred to as *state anxiety*, represents an immediate response that is relatively transitory. The apprehension experienced before a job interview, an important test, or a visit to the in-laws represents state anxiety. State anxiety is often the result of self-doubt, self-criticism, and avoidance behavior. According to Liebert and Morris (1967), state anxiety can be further broken down into cognitive worry, in which the individual imagines negative occurrences, and somatic anxiety, in which symptoms, such as increased heartrate, rapid breathing, muscle tension and sweating, are experienced. The separating of anxiety into two types, trait anxiety and state anxiety (Cattell & Scheier, 1958, 1961; Spielberger, 1966, 1972), has become the most popular method of studying the exercise and anxiety relationship. Only the most recent research has focused on the cognitive worry and somatic anxiety distinction.

Traditional Treatments for Anxiety

For many individuals, symptoms of anxiety usually disappear on their own within a short period of time. For others, these symptoms do not subside on their own. In cases such as these, specific interventions are required to deal with the anxiety.

Treatment for the anxiety states (panic disorder and generalized anxiety disorder) has included psychotherapy, cognitive behavior modification, and drug therapy. In some cases, cognitively learned anxiety can be treated with psychotherapy that attempts to block, restructure, or replace the irrational, incomplete, or poorly formed assumptions that people hold about the sources or potential consequences of events (Dishman, 1986). Recently, a more preventive, self-regulatory approach to anxiety management has been advocated. This technique, known as cognitive behavior modification, attempts to change faulty thought patterns that cause worry or anxiety and substitute new thoughts and behaviors that are incompatible with anxiety (Burns, 1980). Although these techniques have enjoyed reasonable success, their use has been limited by two factors. First, it is difficult to determine if the anxiety is conditioned (cognitively learned) or biologically based. In the former case, behavior therapy will prove effective, but in the latter case it will not. Second, it is very difficult to maintain behavior therapies in everyday life, away from the therapist. For this reason, drugs have been employed as the front-line treatment for anxiety.

Drug therapy for anxiety typically involves the use of minor tranquilizers. The benzodiazepines (e.g., Librium, Valium, Dalmane, Xanax) represent the most common family of minor tranquilizers. Although these drugs provide an effective and fast-acting treatment for the symptoms of anxiety, they also involve some serious disadvantages. First, the benzodiazepines have been widely abused through legal prescriptions as well as on the streets. As recently as 1988, Xanax was the third most frequently administered drug in the United States of America (P. Stern et al., 1990). A second problem involves the finding that prolonged use of the benzodiazepines can produce psychological and/or physical dependence, resulting in severe withdrawal symptoms upon discontinuation (J.W. Long, 1991). Withdrawal typically involves a set of flu-like symptoms, such as nausea, dizziness, fatigue, and restlessness. A final problem with this drug family involves the frequent side effects commonly reported with prolonged use of the benzodiazepines. These side effects typically include skin reactions, dizziness, fainting, blurred vision, headache, nausea, disorientation, depression, agitation, disturbed sleep, and periodic amnesia (J.W. Long, 1991). In spite of these problems, tranquilizers remain popular among users because they produce a welcome tranquility. Their sedative, muscle-relaxing, and anxiety-reducing qualities make them a popular choice for both patient and therapist alike. Clearly, a more positive, less problematic treatment alternative is needed.

The Exercise and Anxiety Relationship

A study by Shapiro et al.(1984) reports that less than one quarter of the 13 million sufferers of anxiety will seek professional help. Of those who do, many of these individuals will be exposed to drug therapy, with its concomitant side effects. This situation highlights the importance of developing self-help skills to prevent or deal with the problem of anxiety. Accumulating research points to exercise as one such strategy.

Before discussing the potential of exercise to impact positively on anxiety, it is important to remedy a misunderstanding that has evolved in the literature. Kerr and Vlaswinkel (1990) have observed that a distinction is often made between acute and chronic exercise effects as well as acute and chronic effects of exercise on anxiety. To avoid this dual distinction, the current book will use the term *acute* to refer to a single bout of exercise, while *chronic* will refer to a prolonged exercise program. In contrast, the short-term effects of exercise will be categorized by psychophysiological correlates as well as state anxiety measures. Long term effects of exercise will be discussed in terms of changes in trait anxiety.

Psychophysiological Correlates

A growing body of research has documented decreased levels of anxiety by means of several objective physiological measures.

Reductions in muscle tension. Low intensity exercise has been shown to be consistently associated with significant reductions in muscle tension as measured by electromyographic (EMG) levels (deVries, 1965, 1968; deVries, Wiswell, Bulbulian,& Moritani, 1981; deVries, Simard, & Wiswell, 1982; Sime, 1977). Similar EMG reductions in muscle tension as measured in the Hoffman reflex, which is an indicator of overall skeletal muscle tension, have also been reported (deVries et al., 1982). These changes have been found to exist for up to one hour following exercise. Until recently, it was believed that moderate- to high-level intensities of exercise did not decrease these measures of muscle tension. New research, utilizing the Hoffman reflex, provides a different viewpoint (Bulbulian & Darabos, 1986). Subjects participating in 20 minutes of treadmill exercise testing at 40% or 75% of VO2 max experienced reductions of 13% and 22% respectively in terms of motor neuron excitability. The authors hypothesized this reduction in overall muscle electrical activity was possibly caused by increases in body temperature paralleling the levels of exercise intensity. It now appears that low, moderate, and high levels of exercise may lead to decreased feelings of anxiety through decreases in muscle tension.

Effects on blood pressure and heart rate. Other studies have documented beneficial effects of exercise on blood pressure (Hannum & Kasch, 1981; Raglin & Morgan, 1985, 1987; Raglin, Turner, & Eksten, 1993) and resting heart rate (Shephard, Kavanaugh ,& Klavora, 1985; Wilfley & Kunce, 1986; Williams & Getty, 1986). An experiment by Raglin and Morgan (1987) compared exercise and quiet rest on blood pressure response in male normotensives and hypertensives. The results of this study support previous research in that reductions in blood pressure were reported after both the rest and exercise conditions. The blood pressure reductions that occurred after exercise were still evident during the 1-, 2-, and 3-hour postassessments. In contrast, quiet rest led to faster and smaller reductions in systolic blood pressure, but the changes lasted only a matter of minutes once the rest condition was terminated. This finding led Raglin and Morgan (1987) to speculate that the quantitative reductions in blood pressure associated with rest and exercise were similar, but there may be qualitative differences between the two conditions. If this finding could be consistently replicated, it would suggest that exercise has greater anxiolytic value than does quiet rest.

Cortical activation. A final objective measure of the acute exercise and anxiety relationship involves the use of an electroencephalogram. It is generally accepted that the presence of EEG alpha brain waves reflect decreased cortical activation. For this reason, researchers have interpreted the post-exercise increase in EEG alpha activity as indicative of a relaxation response or anxiety reduction (Boutcher, 1986; Boutcher & Landers, 1988; Daugherty, Fernhall,& McCanne, 1987; Farmer, Olewine,& Comer, 1978; Kamp & Troost, 1978; J. Weiss, Singh,& Yeudall, 1983). These transient increases in alpha brain wave activity have been documented after submaximal and maximal efforts on cycle ergometers (Farmer et al., 1978). Brain waves have also been found to become more synchronous across hemispheres both during and following submaximal treadmill running (Daniels & Fernhall, 1984; Fernhall & Daniels, 1984) and stationary cycling at 40% to 60% maximum (J. Weiss et al., 1983). This tranquilizing effect of exercise appears specific to skeletal muscle, but is not related to fatigue (Balog, 1983; deVries, 1968; deVries et al., 1982).

Psychometric Measurement: State Anxiety

Whereas these studies portray the potential of exercise in relieving objectively measured symptoms of tension, even greater attention has been focused on the relationship between exercise and psychometrically measured symptoms of anxiety. The acute and chronic effects of exercise on anxiety have been measured psychometrically using the state anxiety scale from the State-Trait Anxiety Inventory (STAI) (Spielberger, Gorsuch, & Lushene, 1970) and the Profile of Mood States (McNair et al., 1971). Both instruments measure "how you feel right now" aspects of anxiety. The majority of studies employ the state anxiety scale due to its specificity and ease of administration.

Types of Exercise Associated With Anxiety Reduction

Research continues to accumulate suggesting that state anxiety is significantly reduced by acute or chronic participation in exercises, such as running (Berger & Owen, 1987, 1988; Blumenthal, Williams, Needels, & Wallace, 1982; Fremont & Craighead, 1987; Griffith, 1984; Long, 1984; O'Connor, Carda, & Graf, 1991; Palmer, 1985; Raglin & Morgan, 1987; Rejeski, Hardy, & Shaw, 1991; Seeman, 1987; C.B. Taylor, Houston-Miller, Ahn, Haskell, & DeBusk, 1986), walking (Blumenthal et al., 1982; B. Long, 1984; Palmer, 1985; T.W. Pierce et al., 1993; Sexton et al., 1989; Steptoe, Moses, Edwards, & Mathews, 1993), cycling (Caruso, Dzewaltowski, Gill, & McElroy, 1990; Felts, 1984, 1989; Griffith, 1984; Otto, 1990; Raglin & Morgan, 1987; Roth, Bachtler, & Fillingim, 1990), swimming (Berger & Owen, 1987, 1988, 1992; Raglin & Morgan, 1987), aerobic dance (Crocker & Grozelle, 1991; Topp, 1989), weight training (O'Connor, Bryant, Veltri, & Gebhardt, 1993), leg ergometry (Raglin et al., 1993),and jumping rope (Taxe, 1985).

Prescription Guideline 3.1

Running, walking, cycling, and swimming are the physical activities most often associated with significant improvements in state anxiety. All of these activities are rhythmic, and involve the use of large muscle groups.

No change in state anxiety following acute or chronic running sessions has also been reported (Carl, 1984; King et al., 1989; Labbe et al., 1988; T.W. Pierce et al., 1993; D.L. Roth & Holmes, 1987; Sinyor, Golden, Steinert, & Seraganian, 1986; Smith, 1984).

Research must now attempt to determine if there are qualitative aspects of exercise that impact differentially on state anxiety. Answers to questions such as "what type of exercise is best for reducing participant anxiety?", "are some exercises better than others in terms of their anxiety reducing effects?", and "how hard and how long must we exercise to get the desired effects?", are now beginning to be answered by the research presented in the following sections.

Comparing exercise types. Berger and Owen (1988), utilizing male and female college students, compared swimming, hatha yoga, fencing, weight training, and jogging in terms of their ability to demonstrate reduced state anxiety. The results of this study revealed only hatha yoga to have a significant beneficial effect. No other significant differences were found among the remaining activity modes. A similar study by Sinyor et al. (1986) randomly assigned 38 males to aerobic (jogging), anaerobic (weight lifting), or waiting-list control groups. No between group differences were seen in terms of posttraining state anxiety. Finally, Sexton et al. (1989) reported no significant differences in terms of psychological benefit between walkers and joggers after an 8-week exercise program. The significant reductions in anxiety across different physical activities reported by Berger and Owen (1988) and Sexton et al. (1989) suggest a possible beneficial effect with a variety of exercise modes.

Prescription Guideline 3.2
  Research has failed to identify the "ideal" exercise to reduce state anxiety. It appears that all exercises have the potential for an anxiolytic effect. No differences have been found between aerobic and anaerobic exercises

---

The small number of studies make this speculation tentative at best. Future research should continue to address this issue by focusing on comparisons between (a) different modes of aerobic exercise, (b) different modes of nonaerobic exercise, and (c) aerobic vs. nonaerobic activities. When research of this nature is completed, it is likely that no differences will be found between modes of aerobic exercise or modes of nonaerobic exercise. Significant differences may be found between aerobic and nonaerobic activities, with the aerobic category experiencing the greatest reductions in state anxiety.

Exercise intensity. A recent review by D.R. Brown (1990) has suggested that 15-30 minutes of aerobic exercise at 60% to 90% of maximum heart rate is sufficient to promote significant reductions in state anxiety. Studies utilizing exercise intensities equal to or greater than 60% maximum heart rate (Berger & Owen, 1992; Crocker & Grozelle, 1991; Felts, 1984, 1989; Rejeski et al., 1991; Sexton et al., 1989; Steptoe et al., 1993; Topp, 1989) have all reported significant reductions in state anxiety following exercise. Similar reductions at intensities of 60% VO2 max. or greater have been documented (Berger & Owen, 1987, 1992; O'Connor et al., 1991, 1993; Raglin et al., 1993; Seeman, 1987), although two such studies reported no significant changes (Hannaford et al., 1988; T.W. Pierce et al., 1993). It is interesting to note, however, that similar anxiolytic effects have been reported at exercise intensities of 30% maximum heart rate (Felts, 1984, 1989). Ten minutes of exercise on a cycle ergometer at a mild to moderate workload (50 rpms @ 300kp) has also been associated with significant reductions in state anxiety according to D.L. Roth et al. (1990). Similarily, walking at a comfortable pace has also been associated with lower   subjective anxiety scores (Sexton et al., 1989). The suggestion that exercise must be performed at an intensity exceeding 70% of VO2 max. (Bahrke & Morgan, 1978; Dishman, 1985, 1986; Morgan, 1979a) or age-adjusted maximum heart rate (Andres, Metz, & Drash, 1978; Dishman, 1985, 1986) does not appear warranted in view of recent research.

Prescription Guideline 3.3
   It is not necessary to exercise at high intensity in order to produce significant reductions in state anxiety. Recent research indicates both moderate and low intensity exercises are every bit as effective as more strenuous activity.

Future studies should attempt to address this issue by measuring state anxiety after exercise performed at graded levels of intensity (e.g., 30%, 40%, 50%...80% VO2 max. or age-adjusted heart rate). The latest findings lead this author to believe that aerobic activity at any exercise intensity will be found to decrease participant state anxiety.

Exercise duration. It has previously been suggested, and accepted, that at least 20 minutes of exercise is needed to experience a reduction in state anxiety (Andres et al., 1978; Bahrke & Morgan, 1978; Dishman, 1985, 1986; Morgan, 1979a). Exercise durations of 20 or more minutes have certainly been associated with significantly lower levels of subjective anxiety (Berger & Owen, 1987, 1992; Crocker & Grozelle, 1991; Felts, 1989; B. Long, 1984; O'Connor et al., 1991, 1993; Raglin & Morgan, 1987; Raglin et al., 1993; Seeman, 1987; Sinyor, et al., 1986; Sexton et al., 1989; Steptoe et al., 1993; Topp, 1989). Recent research, however, suggests there is nothing magical about the 20 minute exercise duration. Lowered subjective measures of state anxiety have now been reported following exercise durations as short as 15 minutes (Rejeski et al.,1991), 10 minutes (Roth et al., 1990), and two sessions of only 45 seconds each (Caruso et al., 1990).

> **Prescription Guideline 3.4**
>   Exercise should be conducted for approximately 15 to 20 minutes in order to produce significant improvements in state anxiety. Although even shorter durations have resulted in beneficial effects, too few studies have been performed to allow meaningful generalizations to be drawn regarding exercise durations under 15 minutes in length.

These most recent studies necessitate additional research aimed at quantifying the duration of exercise necessary to produce beneficial effects. To determine the minimum duration needed to reduce anxiety, experimental studies that manipulate exercise within the 0- to 20-minute time frame (e.g., 5, 10, 15, or 20 minutes) are needed. Research of this nature will likely establish that the duration of exercise needed to produce beneficial results will be shorter than originally believed.

The transient nature of the exercise and state anxiety relationship.
The relationship between exercise and state anxiety appears quite transient, lasting only 4 to 6 hours following participation in the activity (Berger, 1984; D.R. Brown, 1990; Dishman, 1985, 1986; Gleser & Mendelberg, 1990; Kerr & Vlaswinkel, 1990; Morgan, 1981; Morgan & Goldston, 1987; Morgan & Horstman, 1976; Seeman, 1987). Seeman (1987), utilizing a sample of male and female adult volunteers, reported significant reductions in state anxiety following a 20-minute session of running were still apparent at 30-minute, 3-hour, and 5-hour follow-ups. It is interesting to note that the transient reductions in subjective state anxiety following an exercise bout appear to last approximately the same length of time as the objective measures of blood pressure (Hannum & Kasch, 1981; Raglin & Morgan, 1987). The effects of exercise on anxiety, therefore, appear to have both physiological and psychological parameters.

> **Prescription Guideline 3.5**
>   Reductions in state anxiety following exercise appear quite transitory, lasting only 4 to 6 hours following participation in the activity.

Future research should employ both measures in an attempt to document the nature of this association as well as the lasting effects of an acute bout of exercise. If it could be ascertained that the effects of exercise on state anxiety last even longer than we currently believe, this information would prove invaluable in establishing the frequency of exercise needed to keep anxiety at an appropriate level in the participant. In essence, exercise would be needed only as often as required to maintain the transient reductions in anxiety. Exercise, when utilized in this capacity, would serve an excellent preventative function.

Population Trends

Although research suggests that exercise is associated with reductions in anxiety in the majority of cases, it is important to consider possible population trends. Significant reductions in state anxiety have been reported in healthy, asymptomatic college students (Berger, Friedman, & Eaton, 1988; Berger & Owen, 1988, 1992; Caruso et al., 1990; Crocker & Grozelle, 1991; Felts, 1984; Griffith, 1984; O'Connor et al., 1991; Raglin et al., 1993; Rejeski et al., 1991; D.L. Roth et al., 1990; Topp, 1989), adults (Blumenthal et al., 1982; Felts, 1989; Fremont & Craighead, 1987; Labbe et al., 1988; B. Long, 1984; Seeman, 1987; Young, 1979), and children (T.P. Smith, 1984). These same anxiolytic effects have been reported in myocardial infarction patients (C.B. Taylor et al., 1986), and halfway house residents (Lion, 1978). It has previously been suggested that the positive effects of exercise on anxiety are typically reported for nonanxious subjects, but are more pronounced for subjects who have clinical elevations in state anxiety (Folkins & Sime, 1981; Morgan, 1979a). The results of this review certainly support the beneficial effects of exercise for healthy, asymptomatic individuals. These positive effects do not, however, appear more pronounced in individuals with clinically elevated (symptomatic) anxiety. Taxe (1985) has reported significant reductions in state anxiety following varied aerobic activities for adults with clinically elevated symptoms. Similarly, Raglin and Morgan (1987) have documented significant beneficial effects for male pharmacologically controlled hypertensives following aerobic exercise. Steptoe et al. (1993) report similar effects for male and female hypertensives. Hannaford et al. (1988), on the other hand, report no significant changes in state anxiety for 25 male psychiatric outpatients following a 30-minute walk/jog program. Finally, an experiment by Cameron and Hudson (1986) compared the effects of aerobic exercise on 71 male and female inpatients suffering from DSM-III (American Psychiatric Association, 1987) defined anxiety disorders with 37 male and female normals. The results of this study indicated a significant increase in state anxiety following exercise for the high anxious psychiatric patients. In this case, the exercise was probably seen by the individual as one additional stressor. These studies by no means support the aforementioned hypothesis (Folkins & Sime, 1981; Martinsen, 1993) that exercise effects are more pronounced for individuals with clinically elevated symptoms of anxiety. Our viewpoint would support Dishman's (1985) claim that the exercise effects may not be as reliable when the anxiety is a symptom of an underlying primary affective disorder.

Effects of Exercise on Regular Exercisers Versus Non-Exercisers

Future studies should document and/or manipulate exercise histories in the patients to determine if the anxiolytic effects of exercise are better for exercisers than for nonexercisers. Nonexercisers would be expected to be more negatively affected than regular exercisers. The Raglin and Morgan (1987) study, which reported significant reductions in anxiety, utilized subjects who were all regular exercisers. It is also important to compare individually determined exercise programs with assigned exercise. It seems reasonable to assume that subjects already suffering from elevated anxiety would see an imposed exercise session as just another form of stressor. A study by Cameron and Hudson (1986) analyzed the occurrence of anxiety symptoms during exercise in 66 patients with DSM-III defined anxiety disorders and 37 normal subjects. Thirteen of the 66 patients and 8 of the 37 normal subjects reported experiencing increased anxiety in association with exercise. The authors used these figures to conclude that approximately 20% of patients with clinical anxiety disorders or normal subjects experience an acute increase in anxiety associated with physical exercise. Cameron and Hudson are quick to point out, however, that these results should not be construed to imply that an ongoing exercise program is not beneficial in reducing anxiety in clinical and nonclinical populations. The results reported refer only to anxiety occurring acutely during exercise. The results were also based on data that were obtained retrospectively. Clearly, a study in which anxiety ratings are collected during graded exercise is needed to verify these early findings.

Exercise Compared to Other Treatment Modalities for Anxiety

Physical exercise compares favorably with other methods used to reduce state anxiety. Acute exercise now appears equally effective to traditional treatment interventions including meditation and/or relaxation (Bahrke &

Morgan, 1978; Crocker & Grozelle, 1991; B.C. Long &: Haney, 1988a; Martinsen, 1993; Morgan, 1979a; Schwartz, Davidson, & Coleman, 1978; E.G. Solomon & Bumpus, 1978; Topp, 1989), cognitive behavioral methods (Berger et al., 1988; Driscoll, 1976; Fremont & Craighead, 1987; Lobitz, Brammell, & Stoll, 1983; B. Long, 1984), or time out therapy which includes quiet rest (D.R. Brown, Morgan, & Raglin, 1993; Crocker & Grozelle, 1991; Raglin & Morgan, 1987; Seeman, 1987). Bahrke and Morgan (1978) attempted to address this issue by randomly assigning 75 adult male exercisers to exercise, meditation, and control groups. The exercise group walked on a treadmill at 70% maximum heart rate, and the meditation group engaged in Benson's relaxation technique, while the control group merely rested in reclining chairs. Results from this study indicated that exercise, meditation, and quiet rest all resulted in significant reductions in state anxiety. A corollary finding indicated that all three groups experienced comparable reductions. Finally, a study by Crocker and Grozelle (1991) reports similar findings with one major exception. These researchers randomly assigned male and female undergraduates to an aerobic dance exercise group, an autogenic relaxation group, or a quiet rest control situation. The findings support the earlier study by Bahrke & Morgan (1978) in that both the exercise and relaxation groups showed significant and comparable reductions in state anxiety. The Crocker and Grozelle (1991) study differed, however, in that the quiet rest control group was not associated with lowered anxiety. This distinction is an important one. If future research continues to support the notion that quiet rest is as effective as exercise and other therapeutic interventions, it will suggest that the effects of exercise and other treatment modalities may be incidental to nontechnical aspects, such as diversion (Gleser & Mendelberg, 1990). If, on the other hand, control and quiet rest conditons do not lead to comparable reductions in anxiety, and exercise continues to be as effective as other treatment modes, then exercise becomes a viable option. In addition, Raglin and Morgan (1987) found that the anti-anxiety effects of exercise lasted longer than was the case with quiet rest. This would suggest exercise involves distraction and something more. A final benefit of exercise concerns the fact that it has been established as a more cost-effective treatment for anxiety (Fremont & Craighead, 1987) than the more traditional interventions.

Exercise and Anxiety: The Latest Findings

The latest research in this area has provided some tentative answers but has also raised some additional questions. A state- of-the-art meta-analytic review by Petruzzello et al., (1991) concluded that (a) no differences existed among types of state anxiety measures, acute or chronic exercise, different exercise intensities, or for when the state anxiety was assessed, 0 to 30 minutes after exercise; (b) no significant differences were found among different types of aerobic exercise; (c) significant differences did exist between aerobic and nonaerobic exercises, with aerobic exercise showing greater anxiolytic effects; (d) significant differences existed between levels of duration of exercise, with 21 to 30 minutes producing greater benefits than exercise of 0 to 20 minutes' duration. It should be noted that the conclusions of this meta-analysis are based on a foundation of research possessing serious methodological problems (Doan & Scherman, 1987; Folkins & Sime, 1981; Gleser & Mendelberg, 1990; Kerr & Vlaswinkel, 1990; Leith & Taylor, 1990; Petruzzello et al., 1991). Although this meta-analytic review quantifies several important issues, it cannot rectify methodological weaknesses inherent in the research. It would indeed be beneficial for future research to perform a meta-analysis only on well-controlled studies employing true experimental designs as defined by Campbell and Stanley (1963). The conclusions derived from studies that adequately control factors with potential to jeopardize internal and external validity would strengthen our understanding of the exercise and anxiety relationship.

Components of Anxiety

Research is now focusing on differentiating between components of anxiety. A study by Rejeski et al. (1991) has examined psychometric confounds of measuring state anxiety following an acute bout of exercise. Following 15 minutes of treadmill running at 75% maximum heart rate, 30 healthy college-aged males were administered eight items of the state anxiety scale (Spielberger et al., 1970) and the AD-ACL Activation-Deactivation Checklist (Thayer, 1985). On the basis of considerable psychological and psychophysiological evidence, two separate but interdependent activation dimensions, energetic arousal and tense arousal, have been identified (Thayer, 1985, 1987). Utilizing these dimensions, results from this study confirmed that state anxiety did in fact decrease following exercise. However, the authors suggested that interpretation of the state anxiety data collected in conjunction with exercise may be confounded by changes that occur during or following exercise. Closer analysis revealed that those items tapping tense arousal decreased with increasing metabolic demands (i.e., exercise), whereas items tapping energetic arousal increased. Following exercise, subjects were reportedly more calm and relaxed. The authors concluded that although state anxiety decreased during the postexercise recovery phase, this variance may be primarily associated with the two items that refer to general states of deactivation, namely calm and relaxed. This would suggest that decreases in state anxiety may only be tracking physiological recovery. A counter-argument for this viewpoint, however, involves the time period preceding the exercise bout. During pre-exercise, subjects' nervousness/worry increased, and they became less calm/relaxed. Analysis of the state anxiety scores, however, revealed no such increases. If the psychometric scores were indeed tracking physiological arousal, one would expect state anxiety scores to parallel the increases in arousal during the pre-exercise time period. Another explanation is that physiological arousal is not a unitary phenomenon. If this is true, the various factors may behave independently. Replication studies are needed to more clearly establish this relationship.

Cognitive Versus Somatic Anxiety

Current research appears to be placing more emphasis upon differentiating between cognitive and somatic aspects of anxiety in the exercise setting, although some researchers feel this distinction is problematic (Landers, 1994; Raglin, 1990). An experiment by Steptoe and Kearsley (1990) evaluated the influence of meditation and physical exercise on cognitive and somatic anxiety, as measured by the Cognitive-Somatic Anxiety Questionnaire (Schwartz et al., 1978) and the Worry-Emotionality Scale (Morris, Davis, & Hutchins, 1981). In this study, the 340 subjects were competitive athletes, recreational exercisers, meditators, and sedentary controls. Results indicated no significant differences between groups in the cognitive and somatic scales of any measure. A more controlled study by O'Connor et al., (1991) utilized the state version of the STAI (Spielberger, 1983) and the Body Awareness Scale (BAS) (Wang & Morgan, 1987) to evaluate the effects of intense running in the presence and absence of interpersonal competition. Ten male and seven females were recruited from a local running club to participate in the study. In the first treatment condition, the subjects ran in an organized 5-mile road

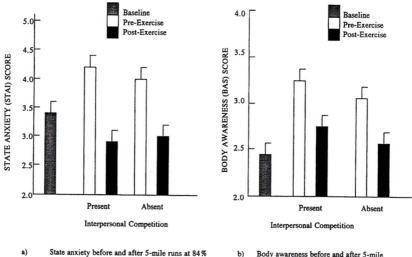

a) State anxiety before and after 5-mile runs at 84 % of VO₂ max.in conditions where interpersonal competition was either present or absent

b) Body awareness before and after 5-mile runs at 84 % VO₂ max.in conditions where interpersonal competition was either present or absent

Figure 3.1. Pre-exercise and post-exercise state anxiety and body awareness scores in the presence or absence of interpersonal competition.
Note. **From "Anxiety and intense running exercise in the presence and absence of interpersonal competition" by P.J. O'Connor, R.D. Carda, and B.K. Graf, 1991, *International Journal of Sports Medicine, 12*, pp.423-426. Copyright © 1991 by George Thieme Verlag Stuttgart. Reprinted with permission.**

race in which they were registered as official entrants. Each participant was asked to run at a self-selected pace, attempting to beat as many other runners in his or her age group as possible. This condition was characterized as involving both intense exercise and interpersonal competition. The second treatment condition involved the same subjects and the same 5-mile course, but was performed one week later. The subjects were asked to run at the same pace as they had run during the road race. This condition was characterized as equal in intensity to the previous treatment, in an environment devoid of competition. The results of this study are presented in Figure 3.1.

Both cognitive (STAI) and somatic (BAS) anxiety were reduced following intense exercise. These reductions occurred in both the presence and absence of interpersonal competition and appeared to be equal in magnitude between the two conditions. These results failed to support the contention of Berger and Owen (1988) that anxiety reductions with exercise are maximized when exercise takes place in the absence of interpersonal competition. Future research should attempt to expand these findings by comparing different types of exercise involving both competitive and noncompetitive conditions. Would these same results occur if team sports rather than individual sports were utilized? Would the competition outcome impact on the anxiolytic effects? A tentative answer to the latter question has been provided by Caruso et al. (1990), who utilized the Competitive State Anxiety Inventory -2 (Martens, Burton, Vealey, Bump, & Smith, 1983) to assess cognitive and somatic aspects of anxiety following competitive success and failure. Twenty-four male and female undergraduates performed a cycle ergometer task across three conditions: noncompetitive, competitive success, and competitive failure. Each condition was performed on a separate day with the order of conditions counterbalanced across participants. The results of this study indicated increases in somatic anxiety in both success and failure conditions, whereas cognitive anxiety increased following failure and decreased following success. This study suggests that competitive state anxiety changes across time and different competitive conditions, supporting the notion that anxiety is a multidimensional concept. These "cutting-edge" studies indicate that the exercise and anxiety association may not be as straightforward as suggested by earlier studies that did not differentiate between components of state anxiety. Morgan and Hammer (1974), for example, reported that anxiety was found to decrease after competition in wrestlers, irrespective of winning or losing. This study, however, utilized a unidimensional measure.

Trait Anxiety

In the majority of cases, the chronic effects of exercise on trait anxiety have been measured subjectively by means of the trait scale of the State-Trait Anxiety Inventory (Spielberger et al., 1970) and the Taylor Manifest Anxiety Scale (J.A. Taylor, 1953). Both tests were designed to assess between subject differences in relatively long-term or lasting aspects of anxiety.

Studies investigating the relationship between exercise and trait anxiety have documented decreases (Eby, 1985; Emery, 1986; Fourman, 1989; Jewell, 1987; King et al., 1993; Kugler et al., 1990; Labbe et al., 1988; B. Long,

1984, 1985; B.C. Long & Haney, 1988a, 1988b; Martinsen et al., 1989a; Nouri & Beer, 1989; Palmer, 1985; Setaro, 1986; Sexton et al., 1989), increases (Stern & Cleary, 1982), or no changes (Abadie, 1987; Berger & Owen, 1987; Carl, 1984; De Geus et al., 1993; Frederick & Ryan, 1993; Goldwater & Collis, 1985; Griffith, 1984; King et al., 1989; T.W. Pierce et al., 1993; D.L. Roth & Holmes, 1987; T.P. Smith, 1984) in trait anxiety. A common feature of these studies is that they all employed aerobic exercises, such as jogging, walking, swimming, cycling, aerobic dance, or "unspecified" aerobic conditions.

Prescription Guideline 3.6
   Chronic participation in a variety of aerobic exercises has been associated with significant improvements in trait anxiety.

Goldwater and Collis (1985) attempted to compare aerobic and nonaerobic activities in terms of their anxiolytic effects. Fifty-one adult males were randomly assigned to one of two experimental conditions. The first group participated in a variety of aerobic activities, including swimming, soccer, and touch rugby. The second group was assigned to a nonaerobic control group. At the conclusion of a 6-week training program, the aerobic exercise group showed improvement in fitness, but only borderline, nonsignificant improvements in trait anxiety ($p=.055$). The control group revealed no changes in either dependent measure. In the Goldwater and Collis study, it is tempting to speculate that if the training program had lasted more than a mere 6 weeks, the improvements in trait anxiety might have reached significance.

Length of exercise program. Support for this viewpoint is provided by Nouri and Beer (1989), who classified 100 male and female adults into one of five jogging patterns. The categories were based on subjects' length of commitment to jogging for at least 20 minutes, three times per week. Advanced joggers were individuals who had jogged for more than 1 year. Intermediate joggers had exercised for 4 months to 1 year, whereas beginners had only participated in the activity from 2 weeks to 4 months. A drop-out group included those individuals who had started a jogging program, then decided to quit. A final group included nonexercisers. The results of this study revealed significantly lower levels of trait anxiety for all jogging groups. Another important finding concerned the observation that the advanced jogging group experienced significantly lower levels of trait anxiety than did subjects in any of the other treatment conditions. This led the authors to conclude that if physical activity is to be effective, individuals must persist over time. An obvious shortcoming of this study involves the nonrandom assignment of subjects to groups and of groups to conditions. It is not possible to infer causation due to the possibility that the groups may have differed in their initial levels of trait anxiety. A natural extension of this study would be to assign subjects randomly to the same treatment conditions, then experimentally manipulate their length of involvement in a jogging program. This would enable the researcher to establish the length of time necessary to produce significant results.

This issue can also be addressed, to a lesser degree, by examining completed research. Training programs have ranged in length from 4 weeks (Palmer, 1985) to 9 months (Fourman, 1989). The majority of studies utilized training programs of 9 weeks or longer.

Prescription Guideline 3.7
  It appears that exercise programs must equal or exceed 9 weeks in order to impact positively on the participant's trait anxiety. Because trait anxiety is a relatively stable psychological construct, longer term programs are probably necessary to produce beneficial outcomes.

Research also exists, however, that documents significant reductions in trait anxiety following exercise programs of 8 week (Kugler et al., 1990; B.C. Long & Haney, 1988a; Martinsen et al., 1989a; Sexton et al., 1989), 6-week (Eby, 1985; Labbe et al., 1988), and 4-week (Palmer, 1985) durations. It would thus appear that short term exercise programs also have potential to impact on trait anxiety.

Exercise frequency. In terms of exercise frequency, most completed studies required exercise to be performed three times per week (Fourman, 1989; King et al., 1993; B. Long, 1984; B.C. Long & Haney, 1988a; Martinsen et al., 1989a; Nouri & Beer, 1989). Two notable exceptions (Goldwater & Collis, 1985; King et al., 1989) involving exercise frequencies of five times per week reported no significant changes in trait anxiety. A possible explanation for this finding is that if exercise is performed too frequently, it may become a stressor in itself, therefore losing its anxiolytic effects.

> **Prescription Guideline 3.8**
> A synthesis of related research suggests exercise must be performed a minimum of three times per week to reduce a participant's trait anxiety.

Not a single study was located that manipulated exercise frequency in an attempt to determine how many days a week a participant must exercise to obtain beneficial effects. Research of this nature would be of significant value to the exercise practitioner.

Exercise intensity. Of similar interest is the question of exercise intensity and duration. Surprisingly, the majority of studies investigating the relationship between exercise and trait anxiety do not document exercise intensities. Of those that do, three report significant reductions (Kugler et al., 1990; Palmer, 1985; Sexton et al., 1989), whereas five report no changes (Abadie, 1987; De Geus et al., 1993; King et al., 1989; T.W. Pierce et al., 1993; D.L. Roth & Holmes, 1987). In all cases, exercise intensities of 60% to 80% (VO2max. or maximum heart rates) were utilized.

> **Prescription Guideline 3.9**
> A paucity of relevant research makes it impossible to make generalizations regarding the relationship between exercise intensity and trait anxiety. For safety reasons, mild to moderate intensities are recommended for the participant.

Clearly, future research must carefully document this information so that replication studies may be performed, and more meaningful conclusions may be generated. Specific studies comparing high- and low- intensity exercises will probably reveal no difference in terms of an anxiolytic effect.

Exercise duration. A final exercise consideration involves the length of time of each exercise bout. All studies reviewed involved exercise sessions of 20 or more minutes, with the majority of studies falling in the 20- to 30-minute range. No trends were discernible in terms of exercise duration and anxiolytic effects.

> **Prescription Guideline 3.10**
> Completed research supports the common assumption that exercise must be performed a minimum of 20 minutes to attain beneficial effects on trait anxiety.

It would be of value for future research to test this assumption by utilizing exercise durations of less than 20 minutes to determine if shorter exercise sessions could produce similar reductions in trait anxiety over the same time period. The limited research available to date would suggest that short duration exercise also has the potential to significantly reduce anxiety in the participant.

Importance of Fitness Gains

Previous research has suggested the importance of documenting fitness gains in research of this nature (Doan & Scherman, 1987; Leith & Taylor, 1990; Thompson & Marten, 1984). Indeed, the majority of studies reporting fitness gains also report significant improvements in trait anxiety (Eby, 1985; Emery, 1986; Jewell, 1987; King et al., 1993; Kugler et al., 1990; Labbe et al., 1988; B. Long, 1984; Martinsen et al., 1989a; Palmer, 1985; Sexton et al., 1989). However, improved fitness gains have also been associated with no changes in trait anxiety (Abadie, 1987; Carl, 1984; De Geus et al., 1993; Griffith, 1984; King et al., 1989). In addition, several studies not measuring fitness have also reported significant reductions (Fourman, 1989; B.C. Long & Haney, 1988a; Nouri & Beer, 1989; Setaro, 1986; C.B. Taylor et al., 1986) as well as an absence of beneficial effects (Berger & Owen, 1987; Frederick & Ryan, 1993; Goldwater & Collis, 1985; Griffith, 1984; King et al., 1989). These latter studies are difficult to interpret because we have no way of knowing if changes in fitness actually occurred, had they been measured. Perhaps these researchers mistakenly assumed fitness changes automatically follow from participation in a physical activity.

> **Prescription Guideline 3.11**
> Changes in fitness do not appear necessary for physical activity to reduce trait anxiety, although a trend in this direction is indicated. This may be due to the fact that in order to improve fitness, the program must be conducted for a relatively long period of time. This extra time may allow the exercise to have a cumulative effect on trait anxiety.

Clearly, something apart from, or in addition to, fitness gains is responsible for the positive effects of exercise on this important psychological construct.

Fitness and Psychosocial Stressors

A somewhat tangential line of research has evolved that focuses on the relationship between fitness and reactivity to a variety of psychosocial stressors (Berger, 1994; D.R. Brown, 1990; Landers, 1994; Sime, 1990). This association has been studied utilizing cardiovascular (Clayton, Cox, Howley, Lawler, & Lawler, 1988; Holmes & Roth, 1985; Roskies et al., 1986; Sinyor et al., 1986), physiological (Clayton et al., 1988; Hull, Young, & Ziegler, 1984; Keller & Seraganian, 1984), biochemical (Blaney, Sothman, Roth, Hart, & Horn, 1990; Sinyor, Schwartz, Peronnet, Brisson, & Seraganian, 1983; M. Sothman, Horn, Hart, & Gustafson, 1987), and psychological (Holmes & Roth, 1985; Hull et al., 1984; Roskies et al., 1986; Sinyor et al., 1983; Sinyor et al., 1986; M. Sothman et al., 1987) measures. The results appear inconsistent, with some studies portraying improved reactivity in fit subjects, whereas others reveal no changes. D.R. Brown (1990) attributes these inconsistencies to the fact that research has employed a wide variety of stressors as well as dependent measures of reactivity. However, a meta-analytic review by Crews and Landers (1987) addresses these specific issues and concludes that "aerobically fit subjects had a reduced psychosocial stress response compared to either control group or baseline values" (p. 114). It would thus appear that fit individuals are at an advantage in dealing with a variety of psychosocial stressors.

Individual Differences and Psychophysiological Reactivity

It has also been suggested that individual differences may influence psychophysiological reactivity to stress, thereby resulting in differential effects of exercise (Balog, 1983; Contrada & Krantz, 1988; deVries et al., 1981; Dienstbier, Crabbe, & Johnson, 1981; Dishman, 1985; Farmer, Olewine, & Comer, 1978; Lake, Suarex, Schneiderman, & Tocci, 1985; Sime, 1977, 1990). Some evidence now exists suggesting that improved physical fitness is associated with a reduction of the Type A behavior pattern (Levenkron & Moore, 1988; Sime, 1990). This finding indicates a potential for exercise to affect both cardiovascular reactivity and the Type A behavior pattern, two separate but related coronary risk factors (Sime, 1990). Conflicting results have been reported by De Geus et al. (1993), however, suggesting exercise does not improve psychophysiologic reactivity.

Significant reductions in trait anxiety have been reported for healthy adults (Fourman, 1989; Labbe et al., 1988; B. Long, 1984; B.C. Long & Haney,

1988a, 1988b; Nouri & Beer, 1989; Setaro, 1986), college students (Griffith, 1984; Jewell, 1987), and elderly adults (Emery, 1986). Studies reporting no changes in trait anxiety have also been reported for similar groups of healthy adults (Goldwater & Collis, 1985; King et al., 1989), college students (Berger & Owen, 1987; D.L. Roth & Holmes, 1987), elderly adults (Abadie, 1987), and children (Carl, 1984; T.P. Smith, 1984). These contradictory findings make it impossible to conclude that healthy asymptomatic individuals benefit significantly from involvement in a prolonged exercise program.

Chronic Exercise and Trait Anxiety in Symptomatic Individuals

Relatively few studies have attempted to ascertain the relationship between chronic exercise and trait anxiety in symptomatic individuals. Raglin (1990) has suggested this lack of research stems from the common notion that exercise may increase anxiety or induce panic attacks in anxiety neurotics. This viewpoint was originally advanced by Pitts and McClure (1967), who demonstrated that lactate infusions commonly resulted in elevated anxiety and panic attacks in anxious neurotics. The suggestion that lactate infusion is analogous to lactate elevations caused by exercise, however, has been shown to be flawed (Morgan & O'Connor, 1989; Raglin, 1990; Raglin & Morgan, 1985), because the metabolic consequences of buffered lactate infusion and intense exercise are not directly comparable. Furthermore, it has been established that in over 70,000 maximal aerobic tests performed at the Cooper Clinic in Dallas, Texas, there was not a single occurrence of a panic attack (Morgan & O'Connor, 1989). Despite this evidence to the contrary, the concern that exercise can induce panic attacks in anxiety neurotics is still prevalent in the field of psychiatry (Barlow, 1988).

Recent research has demonstrated that individuals suffering from clinically diagnosed anxiety disorders can benefit from prolonged exercise programs. Martinsen et al. (1989a) compared the effects of an 8-week aerobic and anaerobic exercise program on trait anxiety in a sample of 79 anxiety disordered inpatients (including panic disorder with agoraphobia). Results from this study revealed increased fitness in the aerobic exercise group and decreased trait anxiety in both groups. The results of this study are portrayed in Figure 3.2. This led the authors to conclude that intensive aerobic exercise, with resulting increases in aerobic fitness, is not necessary for significant reductions in trait anxiety. Similarily, Sexton et al. (1989) have documented similar improvements in trait anxiety following an 8-week jog-

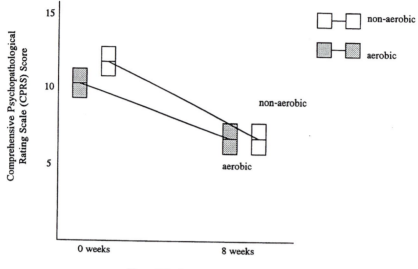

Figure 3.2. Mean Score of the Comprehensive Psychological Rating Scale (CPRS) anxiety subscale, with 95% confidence intervals, comparing the effects of aerobic and nonaerobic forms of exercise on participant anxiety.
Note. From "Aerobic and nonaerobic forms of exercise in the treatment of anxiety disorders" by E.W. Martinsen, A. Hoffart, & O. Solberg, 1989, *Stress Medicine, 5,* p.118. Copyright © 1989 by John Wiley & Sons. Reprinted by permission.

ging or walking program with 52 neurotic inpatients. An interesting implication of this study is that light exercise (walking) and strenuous exercise (jogging) had equivalent psychologic effects. Perhaps even more importantly, the participants rated exercise as more important than either medication or psychotherapy in alleviating their symptoms of anxiety. T.W. Pierce et al. (1993) report conflicting findings with a sample of male and female hypertensives. In this study, no improvements were found after participation in a 16-week walk/jog program.

Finally, significant reductions in trait anxiety have been demonstrated in other symptomatic populations, including the clinically depressed (Eby, 1985), alcoholics (Palmer, 1985), and myocardial infarction patients (Kugler et al., 1990; C.B. Taylor et al., 1986). It, therefore, appears that regular exercise has significant potential for alleviating anxiety in symptomatic populations.

Although it is tempting to conclude that exercise is effective in lowering trait anxiety in both asymptomatic and symptomatic participants, two caveats are in order. First, the results of studies examining the exercise and trait anxiety relationship are more inconsistent than those involving state anxiety. This is hardly surprising when one considers that a prolonged time frame is necessary for exercise to affect the lasting construct of trait anxiety. The occurrence of other life events and common day-to-day stressors may mediate the effects of exercise on this global construct. Second, it is unreasonable to assume that exercise could override the symptoms of a primary affective disorder, such as anxiety neuroticism or any other form of related illness. In cases of this nature, other therapeutic interventions, such as psychotherapy and/or medication, are required. Even so, the possibility exists that although exercise may not be a cure for these individuals, it may result in marginal improvements and prevent the condition from getting any worse.

Quality of Completed Research -- Design Considerations

Before attempting to explain the mechanisms by which exercise may affect anxiety, it is important briefly to consider the quality of research investigating this important relationship. As was done in chapter 2, this will take the form of examining the experimental designs and comparing the results as experiments become more controlled. As a point of reference, the reader is referred to Table 3.1.

Fifty-six empirical studies are summarized in Table 3.1. It is important to note that 41 of the 56 studies (73%) reported significant improvements in anxiety following exercise. In terms of improvement by experimental design categories, 3 of 5 (60%) pre-experimental, 24 of 29 (83%) quasi-experimental, and 14 of 20 (70%) true experimental designs reported significant differences in anxiety following exercise. These numbers indicate a slight tendency towards less observable effects as experimental rigor improves. This finding is consistent with earlier speculations in the literature (Doan & Scherman, 1987; Folkins & Sime, 1981; Leith & Taylor, 1990). On a more positive note, we can state categorically that the weakest experimental designs (pre-experimental) do not inflate our overall percentage of studies reporting significant results. When all the studies are taken together, 73% of them report positive results. This figure exceeds the percentage of pre-experimental studies finding significant improvements. Although the quasi-experimental studies report a higher percentage of improvements than

TABLE 3.1
Empirical Research Investigating the Exercise/Anxiety Relationship

Study	Design	Participants	Controls	Fitness Demonstrated?	Psychological Instruments	Outcome
Abadie (1987)	Quasi-Experimental	Male and female elderly adults	Yes	No	State-Trait Anxiety Inventory, Death Anxiety Scale	No Change
Berger, Friedman and Eaton (1988)	Experimental	Male and female college students	Yes	No	Profile of Mood States	Improved
Berger and Owen (1987)	Quasi-Experimental	Male and female college students	No	No	State-Trait Anxiety Inventory, Cognitive and Somatic Anxiety Questionnaire	Improved
Berger and Owen (1988)	Quasi-Experimental	Male and female college students	Yes	No	State Trait Anxiety Inventory, Cognitive and Somatic Anxiety Questionnaire, Profile of Mood States	Improved
Berger and Owen (1992)	Experimental	Male and female college students	Yes	No	State-Trait Anxiety Inventory	Improved
Blumenthal, Williams, Needels, and Wallace (1982)	Quasi-Experimental	Male and female adults	Yes	Yes	State-Trait Anxiety Inventory, Profile of Mood States	Improved
D.L. Brown (1984)	Quasi-Experimental	Males with chronic obstructive pulmonary disease	Yes	No	Unnamed Instruments	No Change
Cameron and Hudson (1986)	Quasi-Experimental	Male and female psychiatric patients (anxiety)	Yes	No	Symptoms Checklist	Worsened
Carl (1984)	Quasi-Experimental	Male and female special education children	Yes	Yes	State-Trait Anxiety Inventory for Children, Children's Manifest Anxiety Scale	No Change
Caruso, Dzewaltowski, Gill, and McElroy (1990)	Quasi-Experimental	Male and female college students	No	Yes	Competitive State Anxiety Inventory	Improved (success) Worsened (failure)
Crocker and Grozelle (1991)	Experimental	Male and female college students	Yes	No	State Anxiety Inventory	Improved

TABLE 3.1   (Cont.)

Study	Design	Participants	Controls	Fitness Demonstrated	Psychological Instruments	Outcome
De Geus, Lorenz, Van Doornen, and Orlebeke (1993)	Quasi-Experimental	Male adults	Yes	Yes	State-Trait Anxiety Inventory	No Change
Eby (1985)	Experimental	Female depressed adults	Yes	Yes	State-Trait Anxiety Inventory	Improved
Emery (1986)	Experimental	Male and female elderly adults	Yes	Yes	State-Trait Anxiety Inventory	Improved
Felts (1984)	Experimental	Female college students	Yes	Yes	State-Trait Anxiety Inventory	Improved
Felts (1989)	Quasi-Experimental	Female adults	No	No	State Anxiety Inventory	Improved
Fourman (1989)	Quasi-Experimental	Pregnant female adults	Yes	No	State-Trait Anxiety Inventory	Improved
Frederick and Ryan (1993)	Pre-Experimental	Male and female adults	No	No	Taylor Manifest Anxiety Scale	No Change
Fremont and Craighead (1987)	Quasi-Experimental	Male and female adults	No	No	State-Trait Anxiety Inventory, Profile of Mood States	Improved
Goldwater and Collis (1985)	Experimental	Male adults	Yes	Yes	Taylor Manifest Anxiety Scale	No Change
Griffith (1984)	Quasi-Experimental	Male and female college students	Yes	Yes	State-Trait Anxiety Inventory, Life Experiences Survey	Improved
Hammer and Wilmore (1973)	Pre-Experimental	Male adults	No	Yes	Taylor Manifest Anxiety Scale	Improved
Hannaford, Harrell, and Cox (1988)	Experimental	Male psychiatric patients (anxiety)	Yes	Yes	Taylor Manifest Anxiety Scale	No Change
Hayden and Allen (1984)	Pre-Experimental	Male and female college students	No	No	State-Trait Anxiety Inventory	Improved
Jewell (1987)	Quasi-Experimental	Female college students	No	Yes	State-Trait Anxiety Inventory, Profile of Mood States	Improved
King, Barr Taylor, and Haskell (1993)	Experimental	Male and female older adults	Yes	Yes	Taylor Manifest Anxiety Scale	Improved

TABLE 3.1   (Cont.)

Study	Design	Participants	Controls	Fitness Demonstrated	Psychological Instruments	Outcome
King, Barr Taylor, Haskell, and DeBusk (1989)	Quasi-Experimental	Male and female adults	No	Yes	Unnamed Instrument	No Change
Kugler, Dimsdale, Hartley, and Sherwood (1990)	Quasi-Experimental	Male adults with myocardial infarction	No	Yes	MMPI (anxiety scale)	Improved
Labbe, Welsh, and Delaney (1988)	Quasi-Experimental	Female adult volunteers	No	Yes	State-Trait Anxiety Inventory	Improved
Lion (1978)	Experimental	Male and female halfway house residents	Yes	No	State-Trait Anxiety Inventory	Improved
B. Long (1984)	Experimental	Male and female adults	Yes	Yes	State-Trait Anxiety Inventory	Improved
B.C. Long and Haney (1988a)	Quasi-Experimental	Female sedentary adults	No	No	State-Trait Anxiety Inventory, Ways of Coping Checklist, General Self-Efficacy Scale	Improved
Martinsen, Hoffart, and Solberg (1989a)	Quasi-Experimental	Male and female anxiety disordered adults	No	Yes	Comprehensive Psychopathological Rating Scale	Improved
Nouri and Beer (1989)	Quasi-Experimental	Male and female adults	Yes	Yes	State Anxiety Inventory	Improved
O' Connor, Bryant, Veltri, and Gebhardt (1993)	Quasi-Experimental	Female college students	No	No	State-Trait Anxiety Inventory	Improved
O'Connor, Carda, and Graf (1991)	Quasi-Experimental	Male and female college runners	No	Yes	State Anxiety Inventory, Body Awareness Scale	Improved
Otto (1990)	Quasi-Experimental	Female college students	No	Yes	Mood Adjective Checklist	Improved
Palmer (1985)	Quasi-Experimental	Male alcoholic adults	Yes	Yes	State-Trait Anxiety Inventory	Improved
T.W. Pierce, Madden, Siegel, and Blumenthal (1993)	Experimental	Male and female hypertensive adults	Yes	Yes	State-Trait Anxiety Inventory	No Change

TABLE 3.1   (Cont.)

Study	Design	Participants	Controls	Fitness Demonstrated	Psychological Instruments	Outcome
Raglin and Morgan (1987)	Quasi-Experimental	Male adult normotensives and hypertensives	No	No	State-Trait Anxiety Inventory	Improved
Raglin, Turner, and Eksten (1993)	Quasi-Experimental	Male and female college varsity athletes	No	No	State-Trait Anxiety Inventory	Improved
Rejeski, Hardy, and Shaw (1991)	Quasi-Experimental	Male college students	No	Yes	State Anxiety Inventory, Activation-Deactivation Checklist	Improved
D.L. Roth (1989)	Experimental	Female college students	Yes	No	Profile of Mood States	Improved
D.L. Roth and Holmes (1987)	Experimental	Male and female college students	Yes	Yes	State-Trait Anxiety Inventory, Hopkins Symptoms Checklist	No Change
Seeman (1987)	Experimental	Male and female adults	Yes	Yes	State-Trait Anxiety Inventory	Improved
Setaro (1986)	Quasi-Experimental	Male and female adults	Yes	No	MMPI (anxiety scale)	Improved
Sexton, Maere, and Dahl (1989)	Quasi-Experimental	Male and female neurotic inpatients	No	Yes	State-Trait Anxiety Inventory	Improved
Sinyor, Golden, Steinert, and Seraganian (1986)	Experimental	Male adults	Yes	Yes	State-Trait Anxiety Inventory	No Change
T.P. Smith (1984)	Experimental	Male and female children	Yes	Yes	State-Trait Anxiety Inventory for Children	No Change
Stephens (1988)	Pre-Experimental	Male and female adults	No	No	Health Opinion Survey	Improved
Steptoe, Moses, Edwards, and Mathews (1993)	Experimental	Male and female sedentary anxious adults	Yes	Yes	State-Trait Anxiety Inventory	Improved
Taxe (1985)	Experimental	Male and female high anxious adults	Yes	No	IPAT Anxiety Scale, Eight State Questionnaire	Improved

TABLE 3.1   (Cont.)

Study	Design	Participants	Controls	Fitness Demonstrated	Psychological Instruments	Outcome
C.B. Taylor, Houston-Miller, Ahn, Haskell, and DeBusk (1986)	Experimental	Male myocardial infarction patients	Yes	No	State-Trait Anxiety Inventory	Improved
Topp (1989)	Quasi-Experimental	Male and female college students	Yes	Yes	Test Anxiety Questionnaire	Improved
V.E. Wilson, Berger, and Bird (1981)	Pre-Experimental	Male and female adults	Yes	No	State-Trait Anxiety Inventory	No Change
Young (1979)	Quasi-Experimental	Male and female adults	Yes	No	Life Satisfaction Scale, Health Rating Scale	Improved

do the true experimental designs, (83% to 70% respectively), these differences are by no means dramatic. It appears exercise impacts positively on anxiety regardless of experimental design.

Exercise and Anxiety: Suggested Mechanisms of Change

Several mechanisms have been proposed to explain the changes in anxiety following exercise. The two most frequently cited explanations include the thermogenic and distraction hypotheses.

The Thermogenic Hypothesis

It would appear that the thermogenic hypothesis is most suitable to explain the exercise and anxiety relationship. Walking, jogging, and cycling have all been found to reduce physical tension in both clinically anxious and asymptomatic individuals (Johnsgard, 1989). These relaxation effects have been measured in the brain (increased hemispheric synchronization), in the dorsal spine (reflex tests) and in skeletal muscles (electromyograph). Because these same effects can be produced by heating the brain stem or the entire body, deVries (1981) has postulated that the relaxation response to exercise may be linked to the higher body temperatures produced by exercise.

Research indicates that muscle tension levels are indeed reduced following a sauna (deVries et al., 1968). A related study by Raglin and Morgan

(1985) revealed that a five-minute shower at a water temperature of 38.5^C resulted in a significant decrease in state anxiety. Controlled research has also revealed that vigorous exercise results in elevated body temperatures up to 40^C without thermal injury, and this elevation persists for hours after completion of the exercise (Haight & Keatinge, 1973). This increase in body temperature is largely a function of exercise intensity. Canon and Kluger (1983) have shown that rectal temperatures of rats can be elevated by injecting them with plasma extractions from individuals who have just completed exercising. As a result of this finding, the authors concluded that "endogenous pyrogen, a protein mediator of fever and trace metal metabolism during infection is released during exercise" (p. 617).

Conflicting findings regarding the thermogenic hypothesis were reported by Holland, Sayers, Keatinge, Davis, and Peswani (1985). In this experiment, subjects were immersed in warm or thermoneutral water and were asked to perform memory and reasoning tasks. Mood was assessed before and after the experimental conditions, with the results indicating increased irritability in the heated experimental condition. In interpreting this study, however, the authors did not control for the possibility that the cognitive tasks themselves might have been responsible for the increased irritability. For this reason, the conflicting results must be viewed with caution.

These findings, taken in conjunction, have led Morgan (1988) to conclude:

> Because gamma motor activity contributes significantly to muscle tone and because reductions in muscle tension and state anxiety occur following exercise and passive heating, the anxiolytic effects of exercise might be due to a reduction in muscle tension caused by an elevation in body temperature. (p. 111)

The thermogenic hypothesis remains a tenable option for explaining the exercise and anxiety association. Future research needs to examine the effects of exercise on temperature, objective measures, and subjective measures of anxiety taken concurrently. It is also important for studies to compare exercise with passive body heating in terms of their anxiolytic effects. To date, no such studies have been attempted.

The Distraction Hypothesis

The distraction hypothesis originated from the observation that resting quietly in an area free of distractions for 20-45 minutes is associated with significant reductions in blood pressure and state anxiety (Bahrke & Morgan, 1978; Raglin & Morgan, 1987; Seeman, 1987). It has been suggested by Morgan (1988) that exercise involves a component that can also occur in the absence of exercise, namely the passage of time. This "time-out" from anxiety-provoking thoughts and stressors may be responsible for reduced state anxiety (Bahrke & Morgan, 1978). This position has a good deal of intuitive merit. A study by Crocker and Grozelle (1991), however, has failed to replicate these earlier findings. Although both an aerobic exercise group and a relaxation group reported significant reductions in anxiety, a quiet rest control group revealed no changes. Future research must carefully document the exact nature of the time-out period. More specifically, what exactly are the subjects thinking about during this treatment condition, and does this thought content impact on the effects of exercise on anxiety? More replication studies are needed before meaningful conclusions may be drawn regarding the anxiety and quiet rest relationship.

A study by D.L. Roth et al. (1990) has attempted to address this issue. In this experiment, subjects were randomly assigned to exercise versus no exercise treatments, as well as mental task exposure versus no task exposure conditions. In the task exposure condition, subjects were given a variety of distracting cognitive tasks to perform. In the no task exposure treatment, no distraction was utilized. Fifty-seven female college undergraduates participated in the study. An analysis of covariance indicated that exercise, regardless of the task exposure, had an anti-anxiety effect. The authors thus concluded that there is more to the anxiolytic effects of exercise than suggested by the distraction hypothesis. Subjects who exercised but were not distracted still experienced significant reductions in anxiety. Somewhat surprisingly, this study fails to recognize the possiblity that exercise itself may be the distraction. Perhaps it is more difficult to attend to worrisome thoughts when engaged in exercise behavior. Also, the mental stress task could be a form of distraction that acts by diverting subjects' thoughts from real-life stressors. It would be interesting for future research to manipulate thought content to determine differential exercise effects. In other words, what we think of when we exercise may be as important as whether or not we exercise in the first place. A controlled study investigating the effects of positive imagery versus no imagery during exercise may reveal completely different outcomes in terms of their effects on anxiety. A study by Raglin et al. (1993) suggests that distraction may be specific to aerobic exercise and that anaerobic exercise may be less effective and potentially "nondistracting." An empirical study testing the validity of this hypothesis would be worthwhile. Information of this nature would be of immense practical significance to the exercise practitioner. It would also more clearly establish the merit of the distraction hypothesis for understanding the exercise and anxiety relationship.

Summary and Conclusions

Participation in acute or chronic exercise programs appears to be associated with significant reductions in transitory anxiety, as revealed by psychophysiological as well as psychometric measures. These improvements seem to last approximately 1 to 6 hours following the physical activity. Exercise has been demonstrated to be as effective as other traditional treatments in alleviating short-term anxiety. The greatest benefits result from aerobic exercise lasting a minimum of 15 to 20 minutes. Recent research also suggests significant reductions in trait anxiety follow chronic participation in an exercise program. Exercise should be performed at least three times per week to obtain best results. The actual length of the exercise program appears most effective when it equals or exceeds 9 weeks. The results of studies examining the exercise and trait anxiety relationship remain somewhat more inconsistent than do those involving state anxiety. The exact mechanism explaining the exercise and anxiety relationship has not been clearly established. Both the thermogenic and distraction hypotheses remain viable alternatives.

Suggested Readings

Berger, B.G. (1994). Coping with stress: The effectiveness of exercise and other techniques. *Quest, 46,* 100-119.

Berger, B.G., & Owen, D.R. (1992). Preliminary analysis of a causal relationship between swimming and stress reduction: Intense exercise may negate the effects. *International Journal of Sport Psychology, 23,* 70-85.

Brown, D.R., Morgan, W.P., & Raglin, J.S. (1993). Effects of exercise and rest on the state anxiety and blood pressure of physically challenged college students. *The Journal of Sports Medicine and Physical Fitness, 33,* 300-305.

Dishman, R.K. (1994). Biological psychology, exercise and stress. *Quest,*

46, 28-59.

Landers, D.M. (1994). Performance, stress, and health: Overall reaction. *Quest, 46*, 123-135.

Martinsen, E.W. (1993). Therapeutic implications of exercise for clinically anxious and depressed patients. *International Journal of Sport Psychology, 24*, 185-199.

O'Connor, P.J., Bryant, C.X., Veltri, J.P., & Gebhardt, S.M. (1993). State anxiety and ambulatory blood pressure following resistance exercise in females. *Medicine and Science in Sports and Exercise, 25*, 516-521.

Raglin, J.S., Turner, P.E., & Eksten, F. (1993). State anxiety and blood pressure following 30 min of leg ergometry or weight training. *Medicine and Science in Sports and Exercise, 25*, 1044-1048.

Steptoe, A., Moses, J., Edwards, S., & Mathews, A. (1993). Exercise and responsivity to mental stress: Discrepancies between the subjective and physiological effects of aerobic training. *International Journal of Sport Psychology, 24*, 110-129.

Chapter 4

EXERCISE AND SELF-CONCEPT/SELF-ESTEEM

There appears to be good rationale for health scientists to focus on self-esteem as the variable most indicative of emotional adjustment. Both Horney (1950) and Fromm (1956) have documented the underlying feeling of worthlessness characteristic of mental illness. The enhancement of self-esteem represents the primary focus in the development of client-centered therapy (Rogers, 1950) and remains as either an explicit or implicit goal of modern therapies (Wylie, 1979). Research has shown self-esteem to be inversely related to state or trait anxiety in diverse populations (Coopersmith, 1967; Pilisuk, 1963; Rosenberg, 1979). Similarily, acute levels of depression have been consistenly associated with lower self-esteem (Hill, 1968; A. Wilson & Krane, 1980; Wylie, 1979). Low self-esteem has also been linked to problems of neurosis (Angyal, 1951), child abuse (Shorkey, 1980), and adolescent interpersonal problems (Kahle, Kulka, & Klinger, 1980). Conversely, self-concept has been positively associated with the possession of social skills (Crandall, 1973) and the achievement of leadership status (Rosenberg, 1965).

The objectives of this chapter are to (a) introduce the concepts of self-concept/self-esteem, (b) review traditional treatments for low self-concept/self-esteem, (c) introduce the potential of exercise to impact positively on the participant's perception of self, (d) provide a complete research synthesis of empirical studies examining the exercise and self-concept/self-esteem relationship, (e) offer exercise prescription guidelines that can be gleaned from completed research, and (f) discuss the possible mechanisms by which exercise affects this important psychological construct.

Defining Self-Concept and Self-Esteem

Self-concept has been defined by Rogers (1950) as "an organized configuration of prescriptions of the self which are admissable to awareness" (p. 179). Dishman (1986) has expanded the construct to include our ordered awareness of personal experiences, behaviors, and social interactions. He further suggests that our self-concept defines us in comparison with other individuals, as well as our own past behaviors and future goals. A review of literature indicates that early formulations of self-concept tended to emphasize a unitary construct (i.e., a global self-concept) that influenced behavior in a wide variety of settings (Allport, 1937; Mead, 1934; Rogers, 1950). More recently, self-concept has come to be viewed as a multiple domain of self-structure, with specific self-concepts for specific roles in life, such as physical, social, emotional, and academic dimensions (Dishman, 1986; Marsh, 1987; Messer & Harter, 1986; Rosenberg, 1979; Shavelson, Hubner, & Stanton, 1976; Watkins & Park, 1972). Shavelson et al. (1976) have developed a multidimensional viewpoint which maintains that global self-concept is a weighted composite of the more specific self-concepts, as indicated in Figure 4.1.

This model can be seen to portray self-concept as organized and multifaceted, dividing self-concept into academic and nonacademic second order levels. The nonacademic self-concept is further subdivided into social, emotional, and physical self-concepts. Physical self-concept is further subdivided into self-perceptions of physical ability and physical appearance. In addition to these organized and multifaceted features, five additional postulates are fundamental to the model. First, self-concept is hierarchically organized, with lower levels representing situation-specific self-concept, whereas higher levels involve global self-concept. Second, stability is believed to be positively related to the hierarchical level. In other words, situation-specific self-concepts are more susceptible to environmental change, whereas global self-concept is relatively stable. Third, self-concept can be viewed as developmental, with age and experience producing increasingly differentiated conceptions of the self. Fourth, self-concept is evaluative, thus providing a link with self-esteem. Finally, the self-concept is differentiable. This suggests that an individual's nonacademic conceptions are more closely related to each other than they would be to the various academic levels of conception. The major value of this model lies in its ability to demonstrate the multifaceted nature of self-concept.

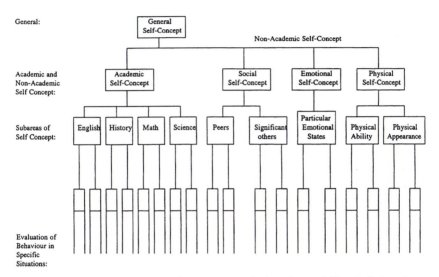

Figure 4.1 Structure of the self-concept, depicting the multifaceted structure for self-esteem in children.
Note. From "Self-concept: Validation of construct interpretations" by R.J. Shavelson, J.J. Hubner, & J.C. Stanton, 1976, *Review of Educational Research, 46,* p. 407. Copyright © 1976 by the Review of Education Research. Reprinted by permission.

Self-esteem has been described as "the degree to which individuals feel positive about themselves" (Gergen, 1971, p. 11), or as a "personal judgment of worthiness" (Coopersmith, 1967, p. 5). It is regarded as the self-concept's evaluative component based on cognitive comparisons and associate affect (Gergen, 1971; Rosenberg,1979). It has been suggested by Wicklund (1975) that because it becomes almost impossible to consider a picture of oneself without experiencing some degree of self-evaluation and/or affect, the terms *self-concept* and *self-esteem* are often used interchangeably. Although this position is accepted, chapter 4 will strive to employ the term *self-esteem* when evaluation and affect are considered, whereas *self-concept* will be used when only self-structure is presented.

Recognizing Problems With Self-Concept/Self-Esteem

It is usually relatively easy to recognize individuals who are suffering from low self-concept/self-esteem. These individuals frequently employ self-deprecatory statements and run themselves down for no apparent reason. They tend to express feelings of worthlessness on a day-to-day basis. They also tend to avoid groups, as well as any form of participatory behavior. Their fear of failure prevents them from trying new activities. In addition, these individuals tend to exhibit several other nonverbal cues, such as poor posture and the avoidance of eye contact. Finally, several special populations have been found to be consistently associated with low self-esteem. More specifically, hemiplegic patients (Brinkman & Hoskins, 1979; Greenwood, Dzewaltowski, & French, 1990), obese people (Collingwood, 1972; Collingwood & Willet, 1971), alcoholics (Palmer, 1985), coronary risk patients (Heinzelman & Bagley, 1970; McGilley, 1987), depressed individuals (Ossip-Klein et al., 1989), and native populations (Scott & Meyers, 1988) have all demonstrated problems with low self-concept/self-esteem. All groups such as these would be likely candidates for problems in this area.

Traditional Treatments for Low Self-Concept/Self-Esteem

Although specific treatments are almost invariably determined by the background orientation of the therapist, two particular treatments appear especially helpful in dealing with problems of low self-esteem. The overall evidence is that group therapy is effective in bringing about positive change (R. Meyer & Smith, 1977; M. Smith & Glass, 1977). In addition, positive outcomes occur most often when the group is composed of members who have at least moderately similar types of problems (R.G. Meyer & Salmon, 1984). The group serves as a testing ground in which clients suffering from low self-esteem demonstrate new behaviors and test new ideas. Group members provide feedback to the individual and often suggest other avenues of response. The setting is believed to promote self-esteem because everyone in the group can occasionally provide help to and express concern for other members of the group. The group is also believed to provide a maintenance function for newly acquired behaviors, as well as a means of entry into new social settings via the friendships formed in the group.

There is also evidence that cognitively oriented behavior therapy can help promote positive self-concept/self-esteem. Extensively developed by Meichenbaum (1977), this form of therapy teaches the individuals to use such things as covert speech or visual imagery to help guide and direct their behavior. With this technique, the client and therapist develop a series of statements or images designed to improve self-image. These positive self-statements and positive images are then practiced until the material becomes second nature. For example, people wishing to improve their self-concept/self-esteem might learn to prompt themselves with self-statements, such as "I'm just as good as the next person" or "today, I'm going to feel real good about myself." An even stronger self-statement, such as "I am a worthwhile individual with a lot to offer," is another example of a self-statement that could be repeated over and over throughout the day. There is a good deal of evidence that how we think determines how we feel (Burns, 1980). With self-statement thoughts such as these, there is a good chance that improved self-esteem will result. As an alternative technique, the client may be taught to use positive visual imagery to improve self-concept. The use of imagery basically involves seeing a picture "through your mind's eye." For example, a person could learn to see a mental picture of him or herself walking confidently down the street, feeling wonderful. More specifically, the client may isolate a problematic occurrence, such as relating with a parent, then develop a "mental movie" of this situation in which the outcome is positive. The client is also encouraged to experience the good feeling that would accompany such an exchange. The main idea is that these positive self-statements and positive imagery become internalized as a way of thinking, elevating the person's self-concept/self-esteem. Cognitive behavior therapy apparently promotes a positive self-image because it promotes feelings of mastery and competence (Kendall & Branswell, 1982). To be effective, these techniques must be practiced regularly.

The Exercise and Self-Concept/Self-Esteem Relationship

Self-esteem has been identified as the variable with the greatest potential to reflect psychological benefit gained from regular exercise (Folkins & Sime, 1981; J.R. Hughes, 1984; Sonstroem & Morgan, 1989). Because body image has been found to be intimately connected to self-image (Berscheid, Walster, & Bohrnstedt, 1973; S. Fisher & Cleveland,

1968; Hamachek, 1987; Secord & Jourard, 1953; Zion, 1965), it is not surprising to find that when one's body image and body functioning improve through physical activity, there is frequently an improvement in one's self-image as well. For example, in an earlier review of research in this area, Layman (1974) noted that "of seven studies involving tests of self-concept before and after a physical development program, four reported improvement in self-concept or body image...and three reported no significant change" (p. 43). Similarily, a review by Sonstroem (1984) focused on 16 studies investigating the causal effect of exercise on self-esteem change in adults and concluded that participation in exercise programs appears to be associated with improved self-esteem scores. A more recent study by Gleser and Mendelberg (1990) reviewed 14 exercise and self-esteem articles and arrived at a similar conclusion. A major problem with these reviews is that they have omitted information concerning specific aspects of the exercise program. It seems reasonable to assume that the mode of physical activity, as well as the frequency, intensity, and duration of exercise, may be important factors in considering the exercise and self-concept/self-esteem relationship. These factors will now be examined within the context of completed research.

Types of Exercise Associated With Changes in Self-Concept

A wide range of physical activities have been investigated in terms of their potential to impact on self-concept/self-esteem. Significant improvements have been reported following participation in running (Bosscher, 1993; E.Y. Brown, Morrow, & Livingston, 1982; Collingwood, 1972; Collingwood & Willet, 1971; Desharnais, Jobin, Cote, Levesque, & Godin, 1993; Hanson & Nedde, 1974; Henning, 1987; Jasnoski & Holmes, 1981; Jeffers, 1977; Joesting & Clance, 1979; King et al., 1989; McGowan, Jarman, & Pedersen, 1974; Ossip-Klein et al., 1989; Saipe, 1978), cycling (Brinkman & Hoskins, 1979), swimming (Collingwood & Willet, 1971; Desharnais et al., 1993), weight training (Jeffers, 1977; Ossip-Klein et al., 1989; Stein & Motta, 1992; L. Tucker, 1983; White, 1974), tennis (Greenwood et al, 1990), basketball (Friday, 1987), as well as a variety of "unspecified" exercise programs (Frederick & Ryan, 1993: Heinzelman & Bagley, 1970; Hellison, 1970; Jasnoski, Holmes, Solomon, & Agular, 1981; Plummer & Koh, 1987; Valliant & Asu, 1985; Wilfley & Kunce, 1986). A substantial number of conflicting results have been reported by studies demonstrating no change in self-concept following running (Davis, 1971; Ford, Puckett, Blessing, & Tucker, 1989; Henderson, 1974; Hilyer & Mitchell, 1979; Leonardson & Garguilo, 1978; C.C. Martin, 1987), cycling (Ben-Schlomo & Short, 1986), swimming (Ford et al., 1989), weight training (Ford et al., 1989; Martin, 1987), tennis (Gussis, 1971), basketball (Bruya, 1977), dance (Radell, Adame, & Johnson, 1993), and "unspecified" exercise programs (Johnston, 1970; Marsh & Peart, 1988; Martinek, Cheffers, & Zaichowsky, 1978; Mauser & Reynolds, 1977; Neal, 1977; Scott & Meyers, 1988).

Prescription Guideline 4.1
Running and weight training are the two types of physical activity most often associated with significant improvements in self-concept/self-esteem. Results appear somewhat inconsistent, with only approximately one-half the empirical studies demonstrating significant beneficial effects.

Although a wide range of exercise modes have been associated with significant improvements in self-concept/self-esteem, in other studies these same exercise modes have been shown to produce no significant changes. In fact, when all the research is examined collectively, only approximately one-half of the studies report significant changes following exercise. Because of these inconsistencies, it becomes important to compare different types of exercise to determine if one particular type of physical activity is superior to others in terms of producing improvements in self-concept/self-esteem.

Comparing exercise types. Studies have only just begun to determine the effects of different types of exercise on self-concept. Experiments (L. Tucker, 1983; L.A. Tucker, 1982a, 1982b) have repeatedly shown that weight-lifting results in significantly greater improvements in self-concept of college males when compared to a nonlifting control group. Ossip-Klein et al. (1989) randomly assigned 40 clinically depressed women to a running, weight lifting, or control treatment condition. Compared to the control group, both exercise treatments demonstrated significant improvements in self-concept as measured by the Beck Self-Concept Scale. The authors further report that "in general, no differences were found between the exercise groups; where the differences did occur, they slightly favored the weight-lifting group" (p. 160). A recent study by Stein and

Motta (1992) provides additional support for the Ossip-Klein et al. (1989) viewpoint. Stein and Motta (1992) employed a pretest-posttest control group design to compare the effects of aerobic (swimming) and nonaerobic (weight-lifting) exercises on self-concept in 89 male and female undergraduates. Self-concept was measured by means of the Tennessee Self-Concept Scale (Fitts, 1964). The results of this study indicated that only the weight- lifting exercise group reported significant improvements in self-concept. Further analysis on the subscales of the Tennessee Self-Concept Scale revealed significant differences between the weight-lifting and control groups in terms of Physical Self, Personal Self, and Social Self scores. No differences were found between the groups in terms of the Moral-Ethical Self subscale or the Family Self subscale. The authors interpreted these findings to suggest that overall self-concept may be tied to the participant's perceptions of his/her body and physical appearance, and that weight lifting has the greatest potential to affect these dimensions.

> **Prescription Guideline 4.2**
>
> It appears that running and weight training are equally effective in improving self-concept/self-esteem. It may be, however, that the appropriate exercise will be dependent on the participant's initial physical appearance. For example, running may be more effective for individuals wishing to lose weight or improve their cardiovascular fitness. Weight training, on the other hand, may be a more appropriate exercise for individuals who are thin or seek to improve their musculature.

Two recent studies suggest that certain qualitative elements of exercise may also impact differentially on self-concept. Marsh and Peart (1988) randomly assigned 137 girls aged 11 through 14 years to one of three treatment conditions. Group 1 participated in an aerobic fitness program involving cooperation. In this condition, participants were required to cooperate in pairs to complete the exercise. The second group also participated in an aerobic fitness program, but the exercises were performed alone with no cooperation among group members. In both conditions, the girls formed teams that competed against one another in terms of the number of repetitions performed by each group. The groups differed, then, in terms of the amount of cooperation required to perform the exercise. A third condition involved recreational volleyball and served as an experimental control. At the conclusion of the 6-week program, only the cooperative group demonstrated significant improvements in self-concept, as measured by the Self Description Questionnaire (Marsh, Barnes, Cairns, & Tidman, 1984). The competitive group actually experienced reduced self-concept at the conclusion of the exercise program. No changes in self-concept were experienced by the control group. The authors concluded that changes in self-concept following exercise may be differentially affected by cooperative and competitive conditions. A study by Caruso et al. (1990) provides additional support for this distinction. Twenty-four male and female college students were assigned to a noncompetition group, a compete-win condition, or a compete-lose treatment. The physical activity involved two repetitions of 45 seconds each on a cycle ergometer. The competition involved counting the number of revolutions performed on the cycle ergometer. In actuality, the experimenters had predetermined whether the participants would win or lose by manipulating the number of revolutions scores reported. In the noncompetition condition, the participants merely performed as many revolutions as possible with no reference given to other individual scores. At the conclusion of the session, participants in the compete-lose condition demonstrated significant reductions in self-confidence as measured by that subscale in the Competitive State Anxiety Inventory (Martens et al., 1983). These two studies, taken in conjunction, suggest that future research must consider the competitive element and the outcome of participation.

Prescription Guideline 4.3
   Recent research suggests the practitioner may be advised to avoid including a competitive element in the physical activity of choice. Competitive conditions, especially those resulting in losing outcomes, appear to have a negative effect on self-concept/self-esteem.

A future research study could combine these elements by employing a 2(competitive vs. cooperative) X 2(win vs. lose) factorial design. The Marsh and Peart (1988) and Caruso et al. (1990) studies would predict an experiment of this nature will reveal main effects for each factor. Studies of this nature will probably indicate that the exercise and self-concept relationship is not as straightforward as suggested by earlier studies not differentiating between competition/cooperation conditions and winning/losing outcomes.

Length of exercise program. The length of exercise programs investigating the exercise and self-concept/self-esteem relationship has ranged from 90 seconds (Caruso et al., 1990) to 18 months (Heinzelman & Bagley, 1970). Exercise programs lasting 8 weeks or less have reported both significant improvements (Bosscher, 1993; Collingwood, 1972; Collingwood & Willet, 1971; Friday, 1987; Greenwood et al., 1990; Hellison, 1970; Ossip-Klein et al., 1989; Saipe, 1978; Stein & Motta, 1992) as well as no improvements (Ben-Schlomo & Short, 1986; Bruya, 1977; Caruso et al., 1990; Davis, 1971; Ford et al., 1989; Henderson, 1974; Marsh & Peart, 1988; Mauser & Reynolds, 1977) in self-concept. Exercise programs ranging from 9 to 12 weeks have also documented improvements (Brinkman & Hoskins, 1979; Desharnais et al., 1993; Jeffers, 1977; McGlenn, 1976; Plummer & Koh, 1987; Valliant & Asu, 1985) and no improvements (Hilyer & Mitchell, 1979; Johnston, 1970; Leonardson & Garguilo, 1978; Martinek et al., 1978; Neal, 1977). Finally, exercise programs of 12 weeks or more document improvements (E.Y. Brown et al., 1982; Frederick & Ryan, 1993; Heinzelman & Bagley, 1970; Jasnoski & Holmes, 1981; McGowan et al., 1974; L. Tucker, 1983) and no improvements (Radell et al., 1993; Scott & Meyers, 1988). It is interesting to note that in both the 8-week or less and 9-to 12-week exercise program length categories, only one-half of the studies are associated with significant improvements in self-concept/self-esteem. In contrast, only one study (Scott & Meyers, 1988) involving exercise program lengths of 12 weeks or greater failed to document significant improvements in self-concept. This observation suggests exercise programs must be performed for at least 12 weeks to produce improvements in self-concept.

Prescription Guideline 4.4

Exercise programs involving 12 weeks or more of participation almost invariably result in significant improvements in self-concept/self-esteem. It appears that the program must be of sufficient length to allow changes in aerobic fitness, body composition, and muscular strength/endurance to occur.

Additional support for this argument can be gleaned from a study by Ford et al. (1989). One hundred and eight female college students took part in aerobic dance, jogging, swimming, life-saving, weight-training, and control treatment conditions. All exercise groups met three times per week for 60 minutes a session for 8 weeks. Exercise intensity was not reported. At the end of the 8-week program, no change in self-esteem was found in any activity group. The authors explained their findings by suggesting that the 8-week exercise program was not long enough to produce changes in participant self-esteem. This question could be addressed by a future experiment that replicates the Ford et al. (1989) study, but utilizes an exercise program length of 12 to 16 weeks. On the basis of completed research (E.Y. Brown et al., 1982; Heinzelman & Bagley, 1970; Jasnoski & Holmes, 1981; McGowan et al., 1974; L. Tucker, 1983), it seems reasonable to predict that these same activities performed over a longer period would be associated with significant improvements in self-concept/self-esteem.

Exercise frequency. The majority of studies reviewed utilized exercise frequencies of two or three times per week. Approximately one-half of these experiments documented improvements in self-concept/self-esteem. It is important to note, however, that when exercise frequencies of greater than three times per week were utilized, the majority of studies reported significant improvements (Collingwood, 1972; Collingwood & Willet, 1971; Hanson & Nedde, 1974; McGlenn, 1976), with only one study (Saipe, 1978) documenting no change. The small number of studies utilizing exercise frequencies greater than three times per week, however, does not allow for meaningful conclusions to be drawn.

Prescription Guideline 4.5

Exercise frequencies of four or more times per week appear most effective in improving self-concept/self-esteem. It is important to note, however, that exercise frequencies of greater than three times per week are not recommended for most participants, especially if initial fitness levels are low. In cases of this nature, it is advisable to employ an exercise frequency of three times per week and maintain the exercise program for a longer period of time. Alternatively, low-intensity exercise, such as walking, may be performed more than three days per week without added risk to the participant.

It is important for future research to investigate thoroughly the question of exercise frequency. If,as suggested by Stein and Motta (1992), self-concept is linked to body image, it may be necessary that exercise be performed more frequently than three times per week to affect physical changes and, concomitantly, body image. It also seems reasonable to assume that exercise must be performed frequently in order to cause physical changes, such as decreased body fat or improved muscle mass. Future research should employ exercise frequencies of four to seven times per week and attempt to measure the actual physical changes associated with exercise, then relate these changes to self-concept/self-esteem scores. Obviously, research of this nature will have to involve subjects who have a relatively high level of initial fitness; otherwise, the increased frequency would be too taxing, and potentially dangerous. Exercises, such as walking, jogging, or swimming would be expected to produce the greatest weight losses, whereas weight-lifting would be associated with improved muscle mass. All of these exercises, if performed frequently enough for a long enough period of time, will likely be associated with improvements in self-concept/self-esteem.

Exercise intensity. Only five of the studies reviewed reported exercise intensities (Ben-Schlomo & Short, 1986; Bosscher, 1993; Brinkman & Hoskins, 1979; Ossip-Klein et al., 1989; Stein & Motta, 1992). Meaningful conclusions cannot be drawn from such a small number of experiments.

Prescription Guideline 4.6
   A paucity of related research prevents the development of a meaningful guideline in terms of the most appropriate exercise intensity to improve the participant's self-concept/self-esteem. In the absence of such documentation, it would be wise to employ only mild to moderate exercise intensities.

It is important that future research begin to carefully document this important information so that replication studies may be performed, and a relationship established between exercise intensity and self-concept/self-esteem.

Exercise duration. A substantial number of experiments did not report the length of each individual exercise session. Of those that did report this important information, an interesting trend is observable. Only one study utilizing an exercise duration of <30 minutes reported improvements in self-concept (Ossip-Klein et al., 1989), whereas two studies employing the same duration reported no change (Ben-Schlomo & Short, 1986; Henderson, 1974). When exercise durations of 30 minutes to 1 hour were employed, three experiments reported significant improvements (Bosscher, 1993; Brinkman & Hoskins, 1979; Friday, 1987), with seven studies documenting no change (Bruya, 1977; Leonardson & Garguilo, 1978; Marsh & Peart, 1988; Martin, 1987; Martinek et al., 1978; Radell et al., 1993; Scott & Meyers, 1988). In contrast, when exercise durations of ≥ 1 hour were employed, the majority of studies reported significant improvements in self-concept/self-esteem (Collingwood, 1972; Collingwood & Willet, 1971; Desharnais et al., 1993; Hanson & Nedde, 1974; Heinzelman & Bagley, 1970; Henning, 1987; Jasnoski & Holmes, 1981; Jeffers, 1977; McGlenn, 1976; Saipe, 1978; Stein & Motta, 1992; Valliant & Asu, 1985), with only four studies documenting no change (Davis, 1971; Ford et al., 1989; Hilyer & Mitchell, 1979; Johnston, 1970). This research suggests that exercise durations of ≥1 hour provide the greatest potential to improve self-concept in the participant. This observation closely parallels the earlier suggestions that higher exercise frequencies and longer exercise programs are associated with greater improvements in self-concept than are lower exercise frequencies and shorter programs. Intuitively, this relationship makes a good deal of sense. When exercise is performed more often, is prolonged, and the exercise program extends for longer periods of time, the potential for physical changes (e.g., weight loss, increased muscle mass) is greatly enhanced.

Prescription Guideline 4.7

Exercise durations of greater than 1 hour are most consistently associated with improvements in self-concept/self-esteem. It is important to note, however, that in almost every instance, the 1-hour time period included both warm-up and cool-down periods. In fact, the actual aerobic or anaerobic exercise sessions usually involved only 20-30 minutes. This is an important caveat, because exercise sessions of greater than 1 hour would pose increased risk of both injury and drop-out.

Previous research has suggested that physical changes have been linked to improved body image, with improved body image impacting positively on self-image (Berscheid et al., 1973; S. Fisher & Cleveland, 1968; Hamachek, 1987; Secord & Jourard, 1953; Stein & Motta, 1992; Zion, 1965). It therefore appears that longer exercise sessions are required to produce improvements in self-concept/self-esteem in the participant. It would be valuable for a future study to employ identical exercise frequencies, intensities, and program lengths while manipulating exercise durations (e.g., 30, 45, 60...90 minutes) to determine the optimal exercise duration required to improve self-concept. Research completed to date suggests that exercise durations $\geq$ 60 minutes will be found to produce the greatest beneficial effects.

Importance of Fitness Gains

The suggestion has been made in previous research (Doan & Scherman, 1987; Folkins & Sime, 1981; Leith & Taylor, 1990; Thompson & Marten, 1984) that it is important to document fitness gains in research of this nature. It certainly seems reasonable to assume that a participant experiencing an objectively measured cardiovascular fitness gain would also experience an improvement in self-esteem. Support for this position can be gleaned from completed research. Wilfley and Kunce (1986) examined the effect of 8 weeks of individually prescribed exercise on the self-concept of 83 male and female adults. The exercise sessions were performed three times per week for 1 hour per session. At the conclusion of the program, the subjects demonstrated significant improvements in fitness (VO2 max.) and self-concept as measured by the Tennessee Self-Concept Scale (Fitts, 1964). A variety of other studies have also documented significant improvements in both fitness and self-concept following exercise (Brinkman & Hoskins, 1979; E.Y. Brown et al., 1982; Collingwood, 1972; Collingwood & Willet, 1971; Desharnais et al., 1993; Friday, 1987; Hanson & Nedde, 1974; Heinzelman & Bagley, 1970; Hellison, 1970; Jasnoski et al., 1981; Jeffers, 1977; King et al., 1989; McGowan et al., 1974; Ossip-Klein et al., 1989; Saipe, 1978; Stein & Motta, 1992; L. Tucker, 1983; White, 1974; Wilfley & Kunce, 1986). An almost equal number of studies, however, have documented fitness gains, but have demonstrated no significant changes in self-concept following exercise (Ben-Schlomo & Short, 1986; Davis, 1971; Folkins, 1976;

Henderson, 1974; Hilyer & Mitchell, 1979; Johnston, 1970; Kowal, Payton, & Vogel, 1978; Leonardson & Garguilo, 1978; Marsh & Peart, 1988; C.C. Martin, 1987; Martinek et al., 1978; Mauser & Reynolds, 1977; Neal, 1977; Palmer, 1985; T.P. Smith, 1984). Taken in conjunction, these studies do not support the notion that cardiovascular fitness gains are responsible for improved self-concept in the participants. This observation is consistent with two recent studies reporting no significant differences between aerobic and nonaerobic exercise in terms of impact on self-concept (Ossip-Klein et al., 1989; Stein & Motta, 1992).

Prescription Guideline 4.8
    Cardiovascular fitness gains do not appear necessary for the participant to experience improvements in self-concept/self-esteem. It is important to note, however, that there are ways to measure fitness other than aerobic power. Body composition, muscular strength/endurance, and flexibility are all components of fitness that remain to be investigated.

Finally, something in addition to fitness gains is responsible for the exercise and self-concept relationship. Recent research by Sonstroem and Morgan (1989), Sonstroem, Harlow, and Josephs (1994), and Sonstroem, Harlow, and Salisbury, (1993) suggests that it is the participant's perception of fitness changes rather than the changes themselves that are responsible for enhancing the individual's self-esteem. More research is needed to adequately test this hypothesis.

Population Trends

The majority of studies reviewed utilized healthy college students, adults, children, and teenagers. Approximately one-half of these studies report improvements in self-concept/self-esteem following exercise. A somewhat different trend emerges when experiments involving special populations are reviewed. Significant improvements in self-concept have been reported following exercise for hemiplegic adults (Brinkman & Hoskins, 1979), paraplegic adults (Greenwood et al., 1990), rehabilitation patients (Collingwood, 1972), coronary risk adults (Heinzelman & Bagley, 1970), obese teenagers (Collingwood & Willet, 1971), elderly adults (Henning, 1987; Valliant & Asu, 1985), clinically depressed female adults (Ossip-Klein et al., 1989), and clinically depressed male and female adults (Bosscher, 1993). Greenwood et al. (1990) studied the effect of participation in the Southwest National Wheelchair Tennis Championships on the self-efficacy of 87 wheelchair-mobile male and female adults. Self-efficacy was measured by means of a situation-specific self-efficacy scale developed for this particular sample and study. At the conclusion of the tennis tournament, participants demonstrated significant improvements in self-efficacy for both tennis tasks and general mobility tasks as compared to a group of 40 wheelchair-mobile non-participants. The authors concluded that participation in wheelchair tennis may increase the competitors' perceptions of efficacy for other physical tasks. It is important to note, however, that the psychological instrument used in this study measures a more labile state that is quite different from the more stable construct of self-concept.

Only three studies utilizing male cardiac rehabilitation patients (McGilley, 1987), native Canadian male and female teenagers (Scott & Meyers, 1988), and male alcoholics (Palmer, 1985) have reported no significant changes in self-concept following exercise programs. Palmer (1985) studied the effects of an "unspecified" aerobic exercise program on a sample of male adult inpatient alcoholics. At the conclusion of the 28-day exercise program, no significant differences were found between the exercise and control groups in terms of self-concept scores as measured by the Tennessee Self-Concept Scale (Fitts, 1964). Contrasting results were reported by Gary and Gutherie (1972), who studied 37 alcoholic male inpatients and found that a 4-week running program resulted in significant improvements in self-concept.

It is interesting to note that only 3 of 13 studies utilizing special populations did not demonstrate improvements in self-concept. J. R. Hughes (1984) has suggested that these positive results with special populations may be a function of the fact that these studies involve subjects with self-concept problems. Support for this position is provided by Hilyer and Mitchell (1979), who studied 120 male college students. Subjects were randomly assigned to a running, running plus counseling, or control group. Subjects were also differentiated in terms of having low versus high self-esteem. At the conclusion of the 10-week program, improved self-esteem was demonstrated only among boys scoring initially low in self-esteem. No changes were reported with boys who recorded high initial self-esteem scores. It is important that future research extend this argument to normal subject populations. For example, a study could stratify male and female college students in terms of pretest self-esteem, then expose them to a prolonged exercise program to see if the two groups are differentially affected. It is tempting to predict, as suggested by Hilyer and Mitchell (1979) and J.R. Hughes (1984), that the greatest gains in self-concept would be experienced by individuals scoring initially low on these dimensions.

Quality of Completed Research -- Design Considerations

Before examining the possible mechanisms with potential to explain the exercise and self-concept/self-esteem relationship, let us briefly consider the quality of research that has been completed to date. Following the same format as employed in the previous two chapters, this will be accomplished by examining the experimental designs and comparing the results as the research becomes more rigorously controlled. Table 4.1 will serve as our reference point for this brief analysis.

Fifty-two empirical studies are presented in Table 4.1. In terms of overall totals, 30 of the 52 studies (58%) reported significant improvements in self-concept/self-esteem following participation in an exercise program. When we look at improvements by experimental design categories, 7 of 10 (70%) pre-experimental, 16 of 26 (62%) quasi-experimental, and 7 of 16 (44%) true experimental designs reported significant improvements in self-concept/self-esteem following exercise. Once again, these figures indicate a tendency towards less observable effects as experimental rigor improves. When one examines Figure 4.1 more closely, however, an alternative explanation arises. Only 3 of the 16 true experimental studies involved special populations. All 3 of these studies (100%) reported significant improvements. The other 13 studies employing the most rigorous experimental design utilized healthy, asymptomatic subjects. Only 4 of these 13 studies (31%) reported improvements in self-concept/self-esteem following exercise. The majority of these studies employed male and female college students, individuals who are unlikely to suffer from low self-esteem. Earlier in the chapter, it was pointed out that only 3 of 13 studies utilizing special populations did not demonstrate improvements in self-concept/self-esteem. This observation suggests that the lower percentage of studies reporting significant improvements in the experimental category may well be a function of the samples studied rather than of improved control-rigor. This alternate explanation

TABLE 4.1
Empirical Research Investigating the Exercise and Self Concept/Self-Esteem Relationship

Study	Design	Participants	Controls	Fitness Demonstrated?	Psychological Instruments	Outcome
Ben-Schlomo and Short (1986)	Experimental	Female sedentary adults	Yes	Yes	Tennessee Self - Concept Scale, Body Cathexis Scale	No Change
Bosscher (1993)	Quasi-Experimental	Male and female depressed in patients	No	No	Rosenberg Self-Esteem Scale	Improved
Brinkman and Hoskins (1979)	Pre-Experimental	Male and female hemiplegic adults	No	Yes	Tennessee Self - Concept Scale	Improved
E.Y. Brown, Morrow, and Livingston (1982)	Quasi-Experimental	Female college students	Yes	Yes	Tennessee Self-Concept Scale	Improved
Bruya (1977)	Quasi-Experimental	Male and female 4th graders	Yes	No	Piers-Harris Children's Self-Concept Scale	No Change
Caruso, Dzewaltowski, Gill, and McElroy (1990)	Quasi-Experimental	Male and female college students	No	No	Competitive State Anxiety Inventory	Worsened
Collingwood (1972)	Experimental	Male adult rehabilitation patients	Yes	Yes	Body Attitude Scales, Semantic Differential, Bills Index of Adjustment	Improved
Collingwood and Willet (1971)	Pre-Experimental	Male and female obese teenagers	No	Yes	Bills Index of Adjustment	Improved
Davis (1971)	Experimental	Male college students	Yes	Yes	Tennessee Self-Concept Scale	No Change
Desharnais, Jobin, Cote, Levesque, and Godin (1993)	Experimental	Male and female adults	Yes	Yes	Rosenberg Self-Esteem Scale	Improved
Folkins (1976)	Quasi-Experimental	Male adults	Yes	Yes	Multiple Affect Adjective Checklist	No Change
Ford, Puckett, Blessing, and Tucker (1989)	Quasi-Experimental	Female college students	Yes	No	Rosenburg Self-Esteem Scale, Body Cathexis Scale	No Change
Frederick and Ryan (1993)	Pre-Experimental	Male and female adults	No	No	Multidimensional Self-Esteem Scale	Improved

TABLE 4.1   (Cont.)

Study	Design	Participants	Controls	Fitness Demonstrated	Psychological Instruments	Outcome
Friday (1987)	Quasi-Experimental	Male teenagers	Yes	Yes	Piers-Harris Children's Self-Concept Scale	Improved
Greenwood, Dzewaltowski, and French (1990)	Quasi-Experimental	Male and Female wheelchair adults	No	No	Study-specific instrument (unnamed)	Improved
Gussis (1971)	Quasi-Experimental	Male teenagers	Yes	No	Tennessee Self-Concept Scale, Body Cathexis Scale	No Change
Hanson and Nedde (1974)	Pre-Experimental	Female adults	No	Yes	Tennessee Self-Concept Scale	Improved
Heinzelman and Bagley (1970)	Experimental	Male coronary risk adults	Yes	Yes	Unnamed Instruments	Improved
Hellison (1970)	Quasi-Experimental	Male college students	Yes	Yes	Rosenburg-Gutman Scale of Self-Esteem	Improved
Henderson (1974)	Experimental	Female college students	Yes	Yes	Self and Body Cathexis Scales, Semantic Differential Self-Concept Scale	No Change
Henning (1987)	Quasi-Experimental	Male elderly adults	Yes	No	Semantic Differential Self-Concept Scale, Personal Orientation Inventory	Improved
Hilyer and Mitchell (1979)	Experimental	Male and female college students	Yes	Yes	Tennessee Self-Concept Scale	No Change
Jasnoski, Holmes, Solomon, and Agular (1981)	Quasi-Experimental	Female college students	Yes	Yes	Self-reported ability estimates	Improved
Jeffers (1977)	Quasi-Experimental	Male and female college students	No	Yes	Self-Ideal, Self-Conceptual Grid	Improved
Joesting and Clance (1979)	Pre-Experimental	Male and female adults	Yes	No	Self and Body Cathexis Scale	Improved for males, No change for females
Johnston (1970)	Experimental	Male college students	Yes	Yes	Q-Sort Technique	No Change

TABLE 4.1   (Cont.)

Study	Design	Participants	Controls	Fitness Demonstrated	Psychological Instruments	Outcome
King, Barr Taylor, Haskell, and DeBusk (1989)	Quasi-Experimental	Male and female adults	No	Yes	Study specific instrument (unnamed)	Improved
Kowal, Payton, and Vogel (1978)	Pre-Experimental	Male and female volunteers	No	Yes	Eysenck Personality Inventory, Profile of Mood States	No Change
Leonardson and Garguilo (1978)	Pre-Experimental	Male and female college students	No	Yes	Semantic Differential Scale	No Change
B. Long (1984)	Experimental	Male and female adults	Yes	Yes	Self-Efficiacy Scale	Improved
B.C. Long and Haney (1988b)	Quasi-Experimental	Female adults	No	No	Self-Efficiacy Scale	Improved
Marsh and Peart (1988)	Experimental	Female children	Yes	Yes	Self-Concept Scale for Adolescents	No Change
C.C. Martin (1987)	Quasi-Experimental	Female college students	Yes	Yes	Tennessee Self-Concept Scale	No Change
Martinek, Cheffers, and Zaichowsky (1978)	Experimental	Male and female children	Yes	Yes	Self-Concept Scale for Children	No Change
Mauser and Reynolds (1977)	Pre-Experimental	Male and female children	No	Yes	Self-Concept Scale for Children	No Change
McGilley (1987)	Quasi-Experimental	Male adult coronary patients	Yes	No	Unnamed Instruments	No Change
McGlenn (1976)	Pre-Experimental	Male teenagers	Yes	No	Other Self Image Questionnaire	Improved
McGowan, Jarman, and Pederson (1974)	Experimental	Male 7th graders	Yes	Yes	Tennessee Self-Concept Scale	Improved
Neal (1977)	Experimental	Male teenagers	Yes	Yes	Coopersmith Self-Esteem Inventory	No Change
Ossip-Klein, Doyne, Bowman, Osborn, McDougall-Wilson, and Neimeyer (1989)	Experimental	Female depressed adults	Yes	Yes	Beck Self-Concept Test	Improved

TABLE 4.1   (Cont.)

Study	Design	Participants	Controls	Fitness Demonstrated	Psychological Instruments	Outcome
Otto (1990)	Quasi-Experimental	Female college students	No	No	Mood Adjective Checklist	Improved
Palmer (1985)	Quasi-Experimental	Male alcoholic adults	Yes	Yes	Tennessee Self-Concept Scale	No Change
Plummer and Koh (1987)	Quasi-Experimental	Female college students	Yes	No	Tennessee Self-Concept Scale	Improved
Radell, Adame, and Johnson (1993)	Quasi-Experimental	Male and female college students	No	No	Body Self-Rating Questionnaire	No Change
Saipe (1978)	Pre-Experimental	Male and female college students	No	Yes	Self-Ideal Conceptual Grid	Improved
Scott and Meyers (1988)	Quasi-Experimental	Male and female native Canadian teenagers	Yes	No	Battle's Culture Free Self-Esteem Inventory, Tyckman's Physical Self-Efficacy Scale, Body Cathexis Scale	No Change
T.P. Smith (1984)	Experimental	Male and female children	Yes	Yes	Piers-Harris Children's Self-Concept Scale	No Change
Stein and Motta (1992)	Quasi-Experimental	Male and female college students	Yes	Yes	Tennessee Self-Concept Scale	Improved
L. Tucker (1983)	Quasi-Experimental	Male college students	Yes	Yes	Tennessee Self-Concept Scale	Improved
Valliant and Asu (1985)	Quasi-Experimental	Male and female elderly adults	No	No	Self-Esteem Inventory	Improved
White (1974)	Experimental	Male college students	Yes	Yes	Tennessee Self-Concept Scale	Improved
Wilfey and Kunce (1986)	Quasi-Experimental	Male and female adults	No	Yes	Tennessee Self-Concept Scale	Improved

would receive support from J.R. Hughes (1984) and Hilyer and Mitchell (1979), who postulate more beneficial effects on self-esteem from exercise when we are dealing with special populations. This argument may also explain why we see fewer overall improvements with the construct of self-concept/self-esteem than we do with depression, anxiety, personality, and mood. If we accept this position, and there appears to be justification for doing so, we can tentatively conclude that exercise appears to impact on self-concept/self-esteem approximately equally across the three design categories.

Exercise and Self-Concept: Suggested Mechanisms of Change

In contrast to the psychological constructs of depression (chapter 2) and anxiety (chapter 3), very little attention has been focused on explaining the relationship between exercise and self-concept. In fact, not a single research study has been found attempting to relate the endorphin, monoamine, or thermogenic hypotheses to improvements in self-concept following exercise. Perhaps the major reason for this observation is that self-concept and self-esteem have not been shown to have biochemical origins. Similarly, the distraction hypothesis appears to be of limited value. In the case of depression or anxiety, a distracting activity, such as exercise, helps to take the participant's mind off disturbing thoughts, thereby making him or her feel better. Self-concept, however, represents more of a psychological trait than a state and as such would be more resistant to change due to a distracting activity. For this reason, more plausible explanations of the exercise and self-concept change mechanism are required.

Self-Efficacy and Skills Mastery

Although the original four mental health hypotheses described in chapter 1 appear to be of limited value in explaining the exercise and self-concept/self-esteem relationship, an additional explanation, referred to as *self-efficacy*, appears promising.

Bandura (1977, 1982) extended the original concept of self-competence to include more specific behaviors. Perceived self-efficacy refers to level and strength of an individual's belief that he or she can successfully perform a given activity. Viewed in this manner, self-efficacy may be viewed as a situation-specific form of self-confidence. According to Bandura, self-efficacy comprises efficacy expectations and outcome expectations. Efficacy expectations ask the question "can I do this particular behavior?" Outcome expectations ask the question "If I do this particular behavior, will I be successful?" In social learning theory, this relationship is referred to as the concept of reciprocal determinism (Bandura, 1977). Self-efficacy expectations not only influence behavior but also are in turn influenced by the success of the behavior. According to Bandura (1977), self-efficacy will influence an individual's choice of activities and settings, the amount of effort expended, and the degree of persistence exhibited at the activity.

Perceived self-efficacy has been used successfully to predict health behaviors such as weight loss (R. Weinberg, Hughes, Critelli, England, & Jackson, 1984), and smoking cessation (DiClemente, 1981; Prochaska, Crime, Lapandski, Martel, & Reid, 1982). Self-efficacy has also been found to predict future exercise behavior in cardiac patients (Ewart, Taylor, Reise, & DeBusk, 1983) as well as the general population (Dishman, Sallis, & Orenstein, 1985).

It is important to note that self-efficacy has been shown to increase as a result of participation in an exercise program (Atkins et al., 1984; Ewart et al., 1983). If exercise can improve self-efficacy, and self-efficacy is a situation-specific form of self-confidence, it is tempting to suggest self-efficacy is the mechanism by which exercise may improve self-concept.

The Exercise and Self-Esteem Relationship: A Proposed Model

Sonstroem and Morgan (1989) have developed a model in attempt to explain the manner in which exercise impacts on self-esteem. This model is presented in Figure 4.2.

This model can be seen to incorporate the seven postulates of the Shavelson et al. (1976) model presented earlier. The model is vertically arranged, with situational self-efficacy at the base of the hierarchy and global self-esteem at the top. This hierarchical arrangement suggests that physical self-efficacy, which is situation specific, is a component of higher level elements, with changes in these lower level elements necessary to produce higher level changes. The horizontal dimension of the model represents order of time, with a pretest separated by the experimental intervention (exercise), then followed by one or more posttests. Sonstroem and Morgan suggest following the American College of Sports Medicine (1991) guidelines specifying a minimal program duration of 15-20 weeks before beneficial training effects are realized. This recommendation is consistent with the suggestion made earlier in the chapter that exercise programs of $\geq$ 12 weeks produce the most benefit in terms of self-concept/self-esteem.

The physical-measures component of the model represents objective data collected from physical tests or fitness measures. The authors suggest using field tests such as Cooper's (1968) 12-minute run-walk, because it provides objective feedback to the participants. Information from these physical measures is used by the participant to formulate physical self-efficacy statements. These statements are situation specific and very susceptible to change. The model portrays how feelings of physical self-efficacy can accumulate and generalize to broader (higher order)

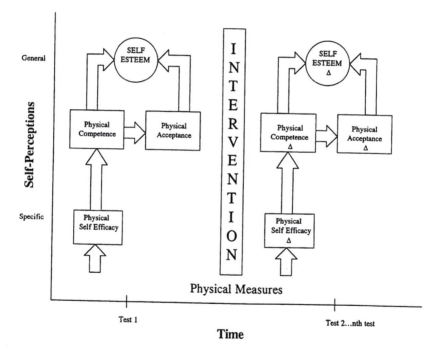

Figure 4.2. Proposed model for examining exercise and self-esteem interactions, depicting vertical arrangement from physical self-efficacy at the base of the figure to global self-esteem at the top of the hierarchy.

Note. **From "Exercise and self-esteem: Rationale and model" by R. J. Sonstroem and W.P. Morgan, 1989,** *Medicine and Science in Sports and Exercise, 21,* **p. 333. Copyright © 1989 by the American College of Sports Medicine. Reprinted by permission.**

feelings of physical competence, which in turn can influence the participant's feelings of physical acceptance. Improved feelings of physical competence and physical acceptance could then influence the more global construct of self-esteem.

The major value of the model rests in its ability to portray self-esteem as a multifaceted construct with potential to change temporally (horizontally) with exercise intervention and hierarchically (vertically) as lower order components accumulate and expand to higher order elements of self-esteem. The model provides a more comprehensive understanding of the exercise and self-esteem relationship and provides a heuristic function for future research. Recent research (Sonstroem et al., 1994; Sonstroem et al., 1993) has added some empirical validation to the Exercise and Self-Esteem Model. In each study, a relatively large percentage of variance was explained by means of path analysis.

Exercise and Self-Esteem: Some Final Considerations

The self-efficacy position appears capable of explaining the exercise and self-concept/self-esteem relationship. It also appears to have theoretical merit. An interesting article by Zeiss and Munoz (1979) addressed the question of why so many forms of mental health treatment are equally effective. In discussing nontreatment variables, they suggested the necessary criteria for success were (a) a rationale providing structure that helps patients believe they can control their own behavior, (b) the teaching of significant skills to the patient, (c) an emphasis on independent use of these skills and personal goal attainment, and (d) attribution of improved mood to the patient's personal skills mastery. Each of these criteria is present in exercise programs. A review by Ledwidge (1980) supports this observation, suggesting that endurance training improves self-respect by means of "the sense of accomplishment that occurs when someone confronts a difficult physical and psychological challenge and overcomes it" (p. 128). Similarly, Shephard (1994) maintains that an increase in self-efficacy, as well as restoration of an internal locus of control, occurs when an individual masters a difficult physical skill. The major implication, of course, is that the participant's involvement must be structured on success, or skills mastery. Exercise practitioners must design physical activity programs to stress the positive and develop skills mastery in small steps or stages. Self-efficacy will be improved if the participant enjoys a series of successes in mastering the exercise behaviors.

Finally, the process of covert behavior modification referred to earlier in the chapter appears to have potential in explaining the exercise and self-concept/self-esteem relationship. The use of positive self-statements and imagery will improve these psychological dimensions by covert positive reinforcement.

Summary and Conclusions

It is interesting to note that the number of empirical studies investigating the exercise and self-concept relationship has dropped off substantially over the past decade. The majority of studies reviewed were conducted prior to 1980. One possible explanation is that interest in self-concept/self-esteem is waning. A more likely alternative is that researchers have focused their attention on specific constructs, such as depression, mood, and state anxiety. The prevalence of clinical and nonclinical problems in these areas has led exercise scientists to explore the role of exercise as a therapeutic adjunct in the treatment of these debilitating disorders.

Approximately one-half of the studies reviewed reported significant changes in self-concept/self-esteem following participation in an exercise program. These results appear quite inconsistent. Recent research suggests exercises that produce observable bodily changes, such as jogging/walking and weight training, have the greatest potential to impact on self-esteem. Exercise programs of more than 12 weeks, with the exercise performed more than three times per week for a minimum of 1 hour per session, have been associated with the greatest psychological benefits. As a caveat, however, a relatively high initial fitness level is required to engage in exercise programs with these frequencies and durations. For this reason, the prescription guidelines offered earlier in the chapter take a more conservative approach. In terms of population trends, it appears that special populations experience more benefit from an exercise program than is the case with the normal population. The self-efficacy/skills mastery hypothesis appears to provide the best explanation of the exercise and self-concept/self-esteem relationship.

Suggested Readings

Bandura, A. (1977). Self-efficacy: Toward a unifying theory of behavioral change. *Psychological Review, 84*, 191-215.

Bosscher, R.J. (1993). Running and mixed physical exercises with depressed psychiatric patients. *International Journal of Sport Psychology, 24*, 170-184.

Caruso, C.M., Dzewaltowski, P.A., Gill, D.L., & McElroy, M.A. (1990). Psychological and physiological changes in competitive state anxiety during noncompetition and competitive success and failure. *Journal of Sport and Exercise Psychology, 12*, 6-20.

Desharnais, R., Jobin, J., Cote, C. Levesque, L., & Godin, G. (1993). Aerobic exercise and the placebo effect. *Psychosomatic Medicine, 55*, 149-154.

Sonstroem, R.J., Harlow, L.L., & Josephs, L. (1994). Exercise and self-esteem: Validity of model expansion and exercise associations. *Journal of Sport and Exercise Psychology, 16*, 29-42.

Sonstroem, R.J., Harlow, L.L., & Salisbury, K.S. (1993). Path analysis of a self-esteem model across a competitive swim season. *Research Quarterly for Exercise and Sport, 64*, 335-342.

Sonstroem, R.J., & Morgan, W.P. (1989). Exercise and self-esteem: Rationale and model. *Medicine and Science in Sports and Exercise, 21*, 329-337.

Chapter 5

EXERCISE AND PERSONALITY

The concept of uniqueness was probably important in the development of early personality research. Questions, such as (a) why are people different?, (b) why do some people behave completely differently than others in the same situation?, and ultimately (c) how am I, as an individual, different from other people?, have generated a great deal of psychological research. This tremendous interest in personality research was quickly adapted to the world of sport and physical activity. A.C. Fisher (1984) has pointed out that well over 1,000 studies were conducted in the so-called "heyday" of sport personality research (the 1960s and 1970s). Most of these studies investigated such concerns as personality trait differences between (a) athletes and nonathletes, (b) successful and less successful athletes, (c) athletes playing one position versus those playing another, (d) team versus individual athletes, and (e) male versus female athletes. Within the field of sport psychology, this sport personality research has remained controversial. Some of the most frequently cited criticisms include (a) a preponderance of atheoretical research, (b) poorly defined independent and dependent variables, (c) poor sampling procedures, (d) failure to use an interaction model, (e) failure to use multivariate data analysis, (f) correlational rather than cause-effect relationships, and (g) failure to account for response distortion (Auweele, DeCuyper, Van Mele, & Rzewnicki, 1993; Carron, 1980; Cox, 1990; Martens, 1975; Morgan, 1980a, 1980b; Rushall, 1973). In addition, Morgan (1980a, 1980b) points out the importance for future research to work with second-order surface traits in personology study. He further maintains that if Rushall (1972) had worked with second-order rather than first-order traits, he would have obtained positive personality results. This viewpoint suggests nonresults of early studies may be a product of either the personality instrument chosen or the statistical technique used to analyze the findings. A final question that still remains inadequately resolved concerns the "change versus gravitation" hypothesis. Proponents of the former position maintain that participation in sport/exercise results in changes in personality traits. The latter argument suggests unique personality traits may gravitate toward exercise, physically active life-styles, or sport. It is important to note, however, that the viability of the gravitational model does not preclude the possibility of exercise positively influencing personality development.

The bulk of these criticisms revolved around what is called the credulous versus skeptical argument(Morgan, 1980b). Proponents of the credulous position maintain that personality testing is useful in predicting athletic success. The skeptical argument viewpoint holds the opposite opinion that personality testing is of little or no value in predicting athletic performance. Although this controversy continues, a moderate viewpoint between these two extremes would seem to describe both the state of this literature and the views of many sport psychologists (Auweele et al., 1993).

The focus of this book is on exercise, not sport participation. As such, our concern is solely with possible effects of exercise on participant personality.

The objectives of this chapter are to (a) introduce the concept of personality, (b) provide an overview of personality theory, (c) outline the current direction of personality research, (d) briefly examine traditional treatments for personality problems, (e) suggest the potential of exercise to impact positively on personality, (f) analyze and synthesize completed research to determine aspects of exercise most conducive to personality improvements, (g) provide exercise prescription guidelines that arise from completed research, and (h) discuss possible explanations for the exercise and personality relationship.

Defining Personality

The Webster Dictionary describes personality as the complex of characteristics that distinguishes a particular individual, or individualizes or characterizes that person in his or her relationship with others. Baron, Byrne, and Kantowitz (1980) suggest that personality consists of an individual's characteristic patterns of behavior that contribute to his or her uniqueness. Finally, a definition by Allport (1937) has withstood the test of time. According to Allport, personality "is the dynamic organization within the individual of those psychophysical systems that determine his unique adjustments to his environment" (p. 48). Regardless of the definition employed, it can be seen that personality represents a multidimensional construct. Over the years, there have evolved several paradigms of personality research. Before moving on to examine the exercise and personality relationship, it is important to consider each of the the major theories of personality research.

Major Paradigms in Personality Research

The term *paradigm* was popularized by Kuhn (1970). A paradigm is really nothing more than a model adopted for an explanatory framework. The use of such a conceptual framework provides a procedure for observing and testing theoretical positions. The model that a researcher adopts will strongly influence his or her general orientation to the study of personality. Although numerous personality theories exist, three specific perspectives are most widely employed. These will be identified as (a) the deterministic perspective, (b) the trait perspective, and (c) the interactional perspective.

The Deterministic Perspective

This paradigm essentially maintains that behavior is determined *for* an individual rather than by an individual. The theories falling under this perspective were strongly influenced by proponents of the 19th-century deterministic-positivistic philosophy that viewed the human as being an energy system (Adler, 1929; Fenichel, 1954; Freud, 1900, 1901, 1917; Horney, 1924; Jung, 1926; M. Klein, 1950). These theorists felt that subconscious processes regulated behavior. They also maintained that the basic dimensions of personality were determined at a relatively early age by means of the resolution of psychic conflicts.

This deterministic perspective is of little value in our understanding of the exercise and personality relationship. Specific and testable hypotheses relevant to physical activity and exercise have not been generated or investigated. Because such a heavy emphasis is placed on subconscious processes, it is very difficult to measure cause-effect relationships between these psychic processes and behavior.

The Trait Perspective

The trait perspective provided a legitimate alternative to the relatively nonquantifiable aspects of the deterministic model. The major assumption of the trait approach is that traits are relatively enduring and nonchanging characteristics that have the potential to predict an individual's behavior in a variety of situations (Allport, 1937). This viewpoint maintains that differences in behavior are due to differences in personality traits (Cattell, 1956; Eysenck, 1960). According to Auweele et al. (1993), traditional trait psychologies share three assumptions: (a) People are cross-situationally consistent; (b) behavior displays a temporal stability; and (c) behavioral manifestations co-occur with the same underlying personality trait. The major concern about this approach is that experience tells us that we behave differently in different situations. Research, in addition to experience, has also raised the issue of the validity of behavior using the trait perspective (Endler & Hunt, 1966, 1968). According to these researchers, personality traits typically explain no more than 10% of the behavioral variability in any given situation. This leaves 90% behavioral variance unexplained. As already mentioned, people do vary their behavior across different situations. If the total range of behavior fluctuations is represented by 100% variance, then 10% explained variance is not particularly illuminating. This finding provides little confidence that behavior can be fully understood by assessment of personality traits. It also avoids the question as to whether these traits are genetic or social in origin. It thus appeared necessary to consider situational factors as well as specific personality traits. Serious questioning of the trait perspective largely originated with Mischel's (1968) book, *Personality and Assessment*. As a result, many personality researchers abandoned trait theory and turned to research based upon behavioral predictability from situational variables.

This situational versus trait controversy of understanding human behavior continued during most of the 1970s. After the polarized dialectic that characterizes such disagreements, a rather old-fashioned but sensible view of interaction between situational and personality determinants of behavior emerged. This viable alternative, called the interactional perspective, acquired a moderate consensus by the end of the 1970s.

The Interactional Perspective

The lack of empirical support for cross-situational stability (a cornerstone of trait theory) has resulted in most contemporary psychologists' adopting a so-called "interactionistic position." The interactional theory attempts to integrate the influence of both the situation and the person upon overt behavior. This model emerged from various social learning perspectives such as J. Rotter's (1954) influential social learning theory, Bandura's (1962, 1965, 1969, 1977) social learning through imitation, and Mischel's (1973, 1977) cognitive social learning. The interactional perspective's most distinguishing characteristic is its emphasis on situational specificity. In other words, individuals regulate their behavior according to the situation (J.B. Rotter, Chance, & Phares, 1972). This viewpoint possesses a good deal of intuitive merit. As characteristics of the situation change, behavioral expectancies are modified. The individual's uniqueness is also emphasized through the concepts of reinforcement histories and reinforcement value (Bandura, 1965; J. Rotter, 1954; J.B. Rotter et al., 1972). An excellent literature review by Auweele et al. (1993) outlines three interpretations of this person-situation interaction. A first variant of this approach is termed *organismic interactionism*, which refers to the reciprocal causal interaction between personality factors and situational characteristics. This viewpoint implies actual behavior is a function of the situation as perceived and interpreted by the individual. In addition, personality characteristics are believed to be the result of past situations (i.e., a social learning perspective of personality). A second variant is termed *statistical interaction*, suggesting the level of one independent variable is a function of the level of another independent variable. In other words, certain personality factors may interact with certain situations, producing a result that is not simply additive. Finally, proponents of dynamic interactionism maintain certain personality characteristics may be responsible for selective exposure to certain situations. This viewpoint closely resembles the gravitation hypothesis presented earlier in the chapter.

This interactional perspective of human personality has become very popular and currently dominates psychological research in this area. It has also been adapted to sport and exercise psychology literature (Martens, 1975; Morgan, 1980b). Morgan (1980b), for example, advocates the interactional position by suggesting the combination of trait and state testing when conducting personality research in sport and exercise. This suggestion appears to have gained little acceptance to date. A notable exception is provided by Morgan et al. (1988), where both state (POMS) and global (trait Anxiety) measures were taken. In this particular study, it was found that global mood and trait anxiety accounted for 45% of the variance in performance of elite male distance runners.

Personology: Three Critical Shifts in Emphasis

The paradigmatic and methodological developments in personology have been well documented by Verstraeten (1987), who outlines three specific changes of theoretical focus. The first shift was from self-description techniques, such as questionnaires and projective techniques, to behavioral assessment. This initial shift may be seen as largely resulting from Mischel's (1968) classic text on personality assessment. A parallel change in research focus is apparent in sport personology, as pioneered by Rushall (1975, 1978). Rushall developed a series of sport-specific inventories to describe units of behavioral information in the sports environment. This approach eschewed trait measures for more situation-specific behavioral assessments and has remained a popular approach to personality research in sport.

A second shift in emphasis has been from interindividual to intraindividual research (Runyan, 1983). This change in emphasis has also been called the nomothetic to idiographic shift, representing an evolution from research on groups to research on individuals. A similar pattern has evolved in sport personology, with more research utilizing single-subject repeated-measures research designs (Rushall, 1975, 1978).

A final shift in emphasis has been from a deterministic model, in which behavior is relatively predictable from personality traits, to a probabilistic model, in which a more flexible view on causality is used. Maddi's (1984) suggestion to move psychology research from actuality to possibility provided initiation in this direction. This viewpoint, through the use of statistics, attempts to determine probability rather than to assume total predictability. The application of this probabilistic model has recently been attempted in sport personology by Bar-Eli & Tenenbaum (1988, 1989), who investigated the probability of a crisis during a basketball game. To date, however, this most recent shift in emphasis has only been applied on a small scale in sport. The reader seeking additional insight into these changes in emphases is referred to a review by Auweele et al. (1993).

Recognizing Personality Disorders

In comparison with the other psychological constructs dealt with in this book, personality disorders are by far the most difficult to recognize. Because they do not reach the psychotic proportions that the schizophrenic, paranoid, and affective disorders often do, they remain far more difficult to diagnose. In addition, individuals with personality disorders usually do not perceive their behavior as disordered or unusual. In fact, they seldom become aware of their pattern unless forced to do so by others, such as a spouse or legal authorities (Millon, 1981). Even so, personality disorders are reported to be among the most frequently occurring patterns in clinical practice (Barrett, 1980). They are also among the most maladaptive, because (a) the psychopathology is pervasive and thoroughly integrated in the personality, (b) the patterns are chronic, and (c) they are very difficult to treat (Barrett, 1980; Millon, 1981). Specific categories include dependent, histrionic, narcissistic, compulsive, passive-aggressive, schizoid, avoidant, borderline, paranoid, and schizotypal personality disorders (R.G. Meyer & Salmon, 1984). Going into detail with these disorders is beyond the scope of this book. Suffice to say it is highly unlikely that we would recognize personality disorders in our clients. A DSM-III diagnosis would require a trained mental health practitioner.

Traditional Treatments for Personality Disorders

The major treatment techniques used today include such diverse approaches as medication, Gestalt therapy, transactional analysis, marital therapy, and behavior therapy. Gestalt therapy resembles the psychodynamic theories in that its emphasis is on becoming aware of oneself and attaining insight through catharsis. It focuses on the here and now, and appears quite effective for dealing with clients who intellectualize their problems without attaining any emotional contact with that problem (Perls, Hefferline, & Goodman, 1958). The Gestalt therapist immediately points out any intellectualization, forcing clients to confront their conflicts more directly, thereby bringing clients into touch with the emotional aspects of their concerns. Transactional analysis (TA) has also proven effective by helping the client conceptualize the disturbed marital interactions that accompany personality disorders. This technique focuses on the "games people play" in relationships (Berne, 1964). By heightening the client's awareness of these relationship games, the disorder is exposed to potential treatment. Marital therapy serves a similar function. Finally, behavior therapy has become a popular treatment technique for personality disorders. Behavior therapy attempts to replace vague and often confusing expectancies with specific guidelines. The use of contracts makes explicit requests for changes in specific behaviors.

The Exercise and Personality Relationship

Some evidence now exists suggesting exercise may also have potential for affecting changes in personality. The majority of research studies investigating this relationship occurred in the 1960s and 1970s, with few studies conducted after 1980. This observation probably reflects the recent trend toward analyzing specific psychological states rather than longer lasting personality traits, which are far more resistant to change. Those studies that have examined the relationship between exercise and the global construct of personality yield conflicting results. Significant changes in personality have been reported in some of the research (Buccola & Stone, 1975; Buchman, Sallis, Criqui, Dimsdale, & Kaplan, 1991; Folkins et al., 1972; Hammer & Wilmore, 1973; Hartung & Farge, 1977; J. Hogan, 1989; Ismail & Trachtman, 1973; Jasnoski & Holmes, 1981; Jasnoski, Holmes, & Banks, 1988; Jones & Weinhouse, 1979; Renfrew & Bolton, 1979; Sharp & Reilly, 1975; Young & Ismail, 1976), whereas other studies report no changes in personality following exercise (Darden, 1972; De Geus et al., 1993; D.V. Harris, 1966; Ismail & Young, 1977; Mayo, 1975; Tillman, 1965; Werner & Gottheil, 1966).

Prescription Guideline 5.1
Research examining the exercise and personality relationship has produced conflicting results. Because personality represents global and relatively stable traits, the positive benefits of exercise appear less consistent across studies.

In these studies, personality was most often measured by means of Cattell's Sixteen Personality Factor Inventory (Cattell, 1965). Dienstbier (1984) maintains that interest in the 16PF is related to the affection most researchers have for psychological instruments derived and validated by factor-analytic techniques. The same author suggests the 16PF is also popular because it assesses factors related to emotional states that seem likely to be affected by exercise.

Elements of Personality Influenced by Exercise

Recent reviews have focused exclusively on reporting changes or no changes in global personality (Doan & Scherman, 1987; Folkins & Sime,

1981; Gleser & Mendelberg, 1990; Leith & Taylor, 1990). This technique is not appropriate because the construct of personality represents a multidimensional concept. For this reason, it is important to consider the effects of exercise on a variety of subscales.

16PF measures of personality change following exercise. The majority of studies investigating the exercise and personality relationship have employed the 16PF, developed by Cattell (1965). This psychometric instrument contains the subscales of outgoing vs. reserved, more intelligent vs. less intelligent, emotionally stable vs. emotionally unstable, assertive vs. humble, happy-go-lucky vs. sober, conscientious vs. expedient, venturesome vs. shy, tenderminded vs. toughminded, trusting vs. suspicious, imaginative vs. practical, forthright vs. shrewd, placid vs. apprehensive, experimenting vs. conservative, self-sufficient vs. group-dependent, undisciplined vs. controlled, and relaxed vs. tense. An overview of studies employing the 16PF reveals that exercise has been associated with participants' becoming more reserved (Hartung & Farge, 1977; Renfrew & Bolton, 1979), intelligent (Hartung & Farge, 1977; Young & Ismail, 1976), emotionally stable (Ismail & Trachtman, 1973; Young & Ismail, 1976), assertive (Jones & Weinhouse, 1979), happy-go-lucky (Jasnoski et al., 1988; Jones & Weinhouse, 1979), sober (Hartung & Farge, 1977), expedient (Renfrew & Bolton, 1979), shy (Hartung & Farge, 1977), trusting (Hammer & Wilmore, 1973), suspicious (Renfrew & Bolton, 1979), imaginative (Ismail & Trachtman, 1973), forthright (Hartung & Farge, 1977; Renfrew & Bolton, 1979), placid (Jasnoski & Holmes, 1981), experimenting (Jasnoski & Holmes, 1981; Renfrew & Bolton, 1979), self-sufficient (Buccola & Stone, 1975; Hartung & Farge, 1977; Jasnoski & Holmes, 1981; Renfrew & Bolton, 1979; Young & Ismail, 1976), group-dependent (Jasnoski et al., 1988), controlled (Jasnoski et al., 1988), and relaxed (Jasnoski & Holmes, 1981; Jones & Weinhouse, 1979; Young & Ismail, 1976). It is interesting to note that only the self-sufficient subscale was associated with significant improvements in more than two studies.

Prescription Guideline 5.2
Self-sufficiency appears to be the personality trait most often associated with positive benefits from exercise. It is possible that adherence to an exercise program results in the participant's feeling he or she is able to successfully complete a project independent of outside help.

The above guideline is consistent with the self-efficacy explanation advanced in chapter 4 (Ledwidge, 1980; Shephard, 1994; Zeiss & Munoz, 1979). This hypothesis could be tested by means of a postexperiment questionnaire requesting this qualitative information. Although most of the other subscales had at least one study reporting improvement, no consistency was demonstrated across the total number of studies reviewed. In addition to this observation, several studies reported no change in any of the 16PF subscales following participation in an exercise program (Darden, 1972; Ismail & Young, 1977; Mayo, 1975; Tillman, 1965; Werner & Gottheil, 1966). The results of these experiments utilizing the 16PF provide only tentative support for the position that exercise impacts positively on a participant's personality.

Other measures of personality change following exercise. Although the 16PF has been used almost exclusively in the exercise and personality literature, several studies have employed different psychometric instruments. A study by Folkins et al. (1972) required a sample of male and female college students to jog two times per week for 30 to 35 minutes a session for 16 weeks. The authors employed the Multiple Affect Adjective Checklist (Zuckerman & Lubin, 1965). At the conclusion of the exercise program, participants experienced significant improvements in anxiety, depression, self-confidence, adjustments, work efficiency, and sleep behavior. A similar study by Sharp and Reilly (1975) employed the Minnesota Multiphasic Personality Inventory (MMPI), developed by Hathaway and McKinley (1967). The MMPI is the most widely used objective inventory of psychopathology in the world and consists of 14 standard subscales. A sample of male college students participated in an aerobic conditioning program two times per week for 45 minutes a session over 14 weeks. At the conclusion of the exercise program, participants scored significantly higher on the personality dimension of ego-strength. None of the other personality subscales were affected by the aerobic conditioning program. A recent study by J. Hogan (1989) utilized a new testing instrument called the Hogan Personality Inventory (HPI), developed by R. Hogan (1986). The HPI measures personality dimensions labeled Intellectance (bright vs. dull), Adjustment (self-confident vs. neurotic), Prudence (conscientious vs. delinquent), Ambition (upwardly mobile vs. anergic), Sociability (extraversion vs. introversion), and Likeability (likeable vs. disagreeable). The HPI has been touted as one of the most carefully constructed and validated of the new generation of inventories of normal personality (Lifton & Nannis, 1988). A sample of 97 adult males

(Navy enlisted) and 35 adult males (police officer applicants) took part in the experiment. All subjects were given a variety of physical tests measuring the fitness factors of muscular strength, endurance, and movement quality. Results of the study indicated a particular personality syndrome is associated with all three fitness factors. J. Hogan suggests people typifying this syndrome are seen as optimistic, energetic, perfectionistic, and competitive.

A recent study by Buchman et al. (1991) eschewed the measure of global personality, focusing instead on a specific personality dimension. The authors employed the Bortner Short Rating Scale, developed by Bortner (1969) to measure overt pattern Type A behavior and the State-Trait Anger Scale (STAS) devised by Spielberger (1980) to measure the intensity of angry feelings and individual differences in anger proneness. The STAS computes three anger variables. "Anger-in" reflects a style of suppressing anger and hostility. "Anger-out" reflects outward expression of anger, whereas "anger-control" involves the extent to which the subject feels he or she is able to retain control over anger and hostile impulses. The subjects chosen for experimentation included 207 male and female first year medical students. Cardiovascular fitness of all participants was assessed by means of a submaximal 5-minute step test adapted from Sharkey (1974). Using stepwise multiple regression analysis, the relationship between the fitness and psychological variables was calculated. Buchman et al. (1991) concluded the most striking and consistent finding was the association between fitness and the anger-in variable. The authors interpret this finding to suggest that improved fitness resulting from regular exercise decreases the quality of angry feelings that are suppressed or internalized. An alternate explanation is that exercise/fitness in some way alters the nature of anger suppression.

As was the case with studies employing the Cattell 16PF, these other measures of personality change following exercise fail to generate consistent results. It appears that exercise has potential to impact on personality, but the specific dimensions of personality most susceptible to change have not been determined.

Types of Exercise Associated With Changes in Personality

Improvements in personality have been associated with participation in exercise programs involving jogging (Buccola & Stone, 1975; Folkins et al., 1972; Hammer & Wilmore, 1973; Hartung & Farge, 1977; Ismail & Trachtman, 1973; Jasnoski et al., 1988; Jones & Weinhouse, 1979; Renfrew

& Bolton, 1979; Young & Ismail, 1976), weight lifting (Darden, 1972; Jasnoski et al., 1988), and aerobic conditioning (Sharp & Reilly, 1975). Other studies, however, report no changes in personality following jogging (De Geus et al., 1993; Ismail & Young, 1977; Mayo, 1975; Tillman, 1965) and cycling (Buccola & Stone, 1975) exercise programs.

Prescription Guideline 5.3
   Jogging is the physical exercise most often associated with significant changes in participant personality. This observation must be interpreted with caution due to the small number of studies utilizing an exercise mode other than jogging.

Comparing exercise types. Very few studies have attempted to determine if one type of exercise is superior to another in terms of its potential to impact on personality. Buccola and Stone (1975) compared jogging and cycling in a sample of older men ranging 60 to 69 years of age. All subjects exercised three times per week for 25-50 minutes per session over the duration of the 14-week program. Although the men self-selected themselves into the two exercise groups, the pre/post design allowed comparison of change over time between groups. The results of the study indicated increased aerobic capacity in each group, but only the joggers changed significantly on any of the 16PF dimensions, becoming more self-sufficient and less happy-go-lucky. The authors concluded there is no obvious reason why the 16PF changes occurred only for the joggers, because both groups improved their aerobic capacity. Closer analysis of the data indicated similar, although nonsignificant changes in the cyclists. In this particular study, jogging was superior to cycling in terms of personality change.

Jasnoski et al. (1988) examined personality changes associated with changes in aerobic or anaerobic fitness. Thirty-nine college females and 63 college males took part in this study. The subjects participated in a 10-week physical conditioning class involving either aerobic (jogging) or anaerobic (weight training) exercise. Aerobic fitness, anaerobic fitness, and personality were measured before and after the 10-week training program. Multiple regression analyses revealed changes in fitness to be associated with positive personality changes (e.g., happy-go-lucky, secure, joining, control), as measured by the Cattell 16PF. A second finding indicated that changes in aerobic fitness were more likely to be associated with positive changes in personality than was the case with anaerobic fitness improvements. The authors concluded the positive changes in personality associated with improvements in aerobic fitness can be attributed to either or both of two factors. A first explanation is that improved fitness enabled subjects to cope more effectively with stress, with the improved coping ability leading to more positive personality changes. A second explanation suggests improvements in aerobic fitness influence the production of brain catecholamines that play a role in determining personality functioning.

Prescription Guideline 5.4
Research has failed to identify one type of exercise as being superior in terms of personality development, although recent findings suggest aerobic exercise may be more appropriate than anaerobic or nonaerobic exercise.

More research is needed that compares different types of exercise on personality changes in the participant. It would be of value for a future study to compare different types of aerobic exercise (e.g., jogging, walking, swimming, cycling) to determine if one activity mode is superior to others. The limited research completed to date suggests all aerobic activities have potential to improve personality in the participant. In addition, it is possible some changes in personality following exercise may be neither beneficial nor detrimental (e.g., introversion-extraversion). This possibility should be addressed in future research.

It would also be interesting to examine the effects of nonaerobic recreational activities (e.g., bowling, volleyball, slow-pitch) on personality dimensions. One would predict that involvement in social exercise of this nature would have potential to improve personality dimensions (16PF), such as outgoing, venturesome, trusting, and experimenting. This hypothesis remains conjecture because no experiment has yet investigated these exercise modes. A final, albeit ambitious study could compare aerobic (e.g., jogging, swimming), anaerobic (e.g., weight lifting, sprinting), and social/ nonaerobic (e.g., bowling, slow-pitch) activity modes to see if personality dimensions are differentially affected. It is tempting to suggest that all three modes would result in improved personality, but the personality dimensions experiencing change may vary across different activity modes. For example, aerobic exercise may cause the participant to become more relaxed, self-sufficient, and emotionally stable. Anaerobic exercise is likely to be associated with changes in tough mindedness, assertiveness, and control. Finally, the social/nonaerobic exercises should lead to improvements in the outgoing, venturesome, trusting, and experimenting dimensions. Once again, these predictions are strictly intuitive, because no data base is presently available to generate related hypotheses.

Length of exercise program. Studies documenting significant improvements in personality have employed exercise programs ranging from 10 weeks (Hammer & Wilmore, 1973) to 4 years (Renfrew & Bolton, 1979). Hammer and Wilmore (1973) studied 53 adult males participating in a 10-week jogging program. Although the study had no control group and did not control for life-style changes, the use of change correlations gives the findings some credibility. At the conclusion of the exercise program, changes in aerobic capacity correlated with becoming more trusting and more shrewd, as measured by the Cattell 16PF. Renfrew and Bolton (1979) also utilized the 16PF on a sample of male adults who jogged five times per week for 40 minutes a session over a 4-year period. Results of this study indicated exercisers were more reserved, expedient, suspicious, forthright, liberal, and self-sufficient than were their inactive counterparts.

The majority of studies reporting positive benefits of exercise on personality employed exercise programs of 3 to 12 months(Buccola & Stone, 1975; Folkins et al., 1972; Ismail & Trachtman, 1973; Jones & Weinhouse, 1979; Sharp & Reilly, 1975; Young & Ismail, 1976).

Prescription Guideline 5.5
Exercise programs must be performed for a minimum of 3 months to impact positively on participant personality. It is likely that even longer involvement would produce the most consistent results.

Because personality involves relatively stable traits, it seems reasonable that exercise programs must be of sufficient length to allow for changes to occur. A future research effort should employ a particular exercise mode, with the frequency, intensity, and duration of the activity held constant, then manipulate the duration of exercise program (e.g., 2 months, 4 months, 6 months,...12 months) in a repeated measures design to determine the time required for exercise programs to impact on personality dimensions in the participant. It seems reasonable to assume that longer exercise programs would be associated with stronger correlations of personality change.

Exercise frequency. The majority of studies reporting positive results required the exercise to be performed three times per week (Buccola & Stone,

1975; Hartung & Farge, 1977; Ismail & Trachtman, 1973; Jones & Weinhouse, 1979; Young & Ismail, 1976), although significant improvements in personality have been reported with exercise frequencies of five times per week (Renfrew & Bolton, 1979), and two times per week (Folkins et al., 1972; Jasnoski et al., 1988; Sharp & Reilly, 1975).

Prescription Guideline 5.6
No differences are discernible in terms of exercise frequency and personality changes in the participant. For this reason, an exercise frequency of three times per week is recommended. This frequency appears as effective as higher frequencies without the added risk of injury and drop-out.

Exercise intensity. In terms of exercise intensity, only two studies (De Geus et al., 1993; Jones & Weinhouse, 1979) reported this valuable information. Jones and Weinhouse required a sample of male and female adults to participate in a running program three times per week for 45 minutes a session at 75% maximum heart rate. At the conclusion of the 12-month program, the participants were significantly more assertive, happy-go-lucky, and relaxed as measured by the Cattell 16PF. In the De Geus et al. (1993) study, a group of male adults exercised at 70% VO2 max. for 1.5 to 2.5 hours per week in a chronic program. Results of this experiment reported no significant personality changes.

Prescription Guideline 5.7
Although only two studies reported exercise intensity, the majority of research employed jogging as the mode of physical exercise. For this reason, it seems reasonable to conclude that these studies probably involved exercise intensities of 50%-75% maximum heart rate or VO2 max., due to the nature of the activity.

Obviously, a relatively wide range of possible exercise intensities exists due to the nature of individual differences, as well as the amount of effort put into the exercise sessions. It would be valuable for a future study to compare exercise intensities in terms of their potential to impact on participant personalities. For example, a multiple regression analysis, looking at correlations between selected personality inventory variables and exercise intensities, would prove invaluable. On the basis of completed research, it is likely that an experiment of this nature will determine different intensities to be associated with personality changes over a prolonged exercise program. The relative degree of change remains to be determined. It is possible that moderate-intensity exercise may be associated with the greatest improvements, because the exercise is intense enough to produce fitness gains, but not so intense as to provide an unenjoyable exercise experience. This hypothesis remains to be tested.

Exercise duration. A final exercise consideration involves the duration of the physical activity. Exercise durations as short as 15 minutes (Hartung & Farge, 1977) and as long as 1.5 hours (Ismail & Trachtman, 1973) have been reported. An experiment by Hartung and Farge (1977) studied a sample of male adult joggers who were jogging at least two miles per day (15 minutes per session), 3 days per week. All subjects had been jogging from 1 to 5 years. Results of this experiment revealed joggers to be significantly more reserved, intelligent, shy, forthright, and self-sufficient than the general population. Another study performed by Ismail and Trachtman (1973) employed a much longer exercise duration, requiring a sample of male adults to exercise for 1.5 hours per session. Ten minutes was devoted to warm-up exercises, followed by 30 to 45 minutes of calisthenics, then supervised running, followed by 30 minutes of recreational activities (e.g., basketball, squash, volleyball, or swimming). At the conclusion of the 4-month program, the participants were shown to have experienced significant improvements in emotional stability and imagination as measured by the 16PF. Whereas the Hartung and Farge (1977) and Ismail and Trachtman (1973) studies employed the shortest and longest exercise durations respectively, the majority of studies reporting positive benefits utilized exercise durations of 40 to 60 minutes (Buccola & Stone, 1975; Jasnoski et al., 1988; Jones & Weinhouse, 1979; Renfrew & Bolton, 1979; Sharp & Reilly, 1975).

Prescription Guideline 5.8
   A review of the literature revealed all exercise durations to be equally effective in promoting personality changes in the participant. For this reason, there appears to be no advantage in exercising longer than 20 minutes, unless the participant is exercising for reasons other than mental health.

Importance of Fitness Gains

The majority of studies investigating the exercise and personality relationship also report fitness changes as a result of the exercise programs. Many of the studies documenting fitness gains have also reported significant improvements in personality (Buccola & Stone, 1975; Buchman et al., 1991; Folkins et al., 1972; Hartung & Farge, 1977; J. Hogan, 1989; Jasnoski & Holmes, 1981; Jasnoski et al., 1988; Jones & Weinhouse, 1979; Sharp & Reilly, 1975; Young & Ismail, 1976), although four such studies report no changes in personality associated with fitness gains (D.V. Harris, 1966; Ismail & Young, 1977; Mayo, 1975; Tillman, 1965). Studies not documenting fitness gains have also been associated with significant improvements in personality (Ismail & Trachtman, 1973; Renfrew & Bolton, 1979), as well as no changes (Darden, 1972; De Geus et al., 1993; Werner & Gottheil, 1966).

> **Prescription Guideline 5.9**
> Completed research is suggestive of a trend towards more positive personality benefits when fitness improvements are documented. It is important to note, however, that body composition, flexibility, and muscular strength/endurance fitness dimensions have not been investigated.

Additional support for this viewpoint can be gleaned from studies that compare subjects with different fitness levels in terms of personality characteristics. Young and Ismail (1976) demonstrated significant personality differences between 14 highly fit and 14 unfit middle-aged adults on seven of the dimensions measured by the 16PF. A similar study by Jasnoski and Holmes (1981) investigated the relationship between initial levels of fitness and personality changes in a sample of 103 college females. Statistically significant differences were found between the high-fit and low-fit subjects, with the high- fit group being more placid, experimenting, and relaxed. More recent studies have also associated higher levels of fitness with decreases in Type A behavior patterns (Buchman et al., 1991) as well as more optimistic, energetic, perfectionistic, and competitive personality dimensions (J. Hogan, 1989). These findings are in contrast to two earlier studies (D.V. Harris, 1966; Mayo, 1975), which did not document differences in personality between fit and unfit subjects.

It is tempting to suggest that more positive benefits of exercise on personality occur when fitness gains are documented because of the time involved in order to bring about changes in aerobic fitness. This time frame would necessitate exposure to exercise over a relatively long time frame. As such, exercise would have more opportunity to impact on the participant's personality. If this is true, it may be that fitness per se is not as important as involvement in a prolonged exercise program. Some support for this argument can be taken from the earlier studies by Ismail and Trachtman (1973) and Renfrew and Bolton (1979) documenting improvements in personality in the absence of fitness gains. Research is needed that compares aerobic and nonaerobic exercises in terms of their effects on participant personality. It is suspected that research of this nature will not establish a cause-effect relationship between fitness and improvements in personality scores.

Population Trends

In studying the exercise and personality relationship, healthy, asymptomatic subjects have been studied in the form of college students (Buchman et al., 1991; Folkins et al., 1972; D.V. Harris, 1966; Jasnoski & Holmes, 1981; Jasnoski et al., 1988; Sharp & Reilly, 1975; Werner & Gottheil, 1966), adults (Darden, 1972; Hartung & Farge, 1977; J. Hogan, 1989; Ismail & Trachtman, 1973; Ismail & Young, 1977; Jones & Weinhouse, 1979; Renfrew & Bolton, 1979; Young & Ismail, 1976), teenagers (Tillman, 1965), and children (Mayo, 1975). Without exception, all studies have employed healthy subjects. It is surprising that not a single study was found utilizing subjects experiencing clinical problems with anxiety, depression, or any other form of mood disorder. Although these symptoms represent emotional states, it seems reasonable to expect these individuals would experience the greatest personality benefits from an exercise program. Because it has already been established that exercise has the potential to impact positively on the psychological states of anxiety (chapter 3) and depression (chapter 2), prolonged involvement in an exercise program may have a cumulative effect and lead to improvements in the more stable traits of personality. Future research could verify this hypothesis by including pre and post personality measures in those studies investigating the effects of exercise on anxiety and depression. If the exercise program is conducted for a long enough period of time, personality traits such as relaxed, happy-go-lucky, and emotionally stable may be positively affected. The use of both state and trait measures in the same study is needed to test this hypothesis.

Quality of Completed Research -- Design Considerations

We saw earlier in the chapter that the quality of research investigating the personality and sports participation relationship has come under considerable scrutiny. It is, therefore, important to examine the quality of research looking at exercise and personality to determine if meaningful conclusions may be generated. We will do this by examining the experimental designs and comparing the results as research control-rigor improves. Table 5.1 summarizes the research that has been completed to date.

In contrast to the plethora of research on the sport and personality relationship, relatively few studies have examined the effect of exercise on personality dimensions. Twenty studies are summarized in Table 5.1. In terms of overall results, 13 of the 20 studies (65%) reported significant improvements in at least one personality subscale. When we look at improvements by design categories, 6 of 8 (75%) pre-experimental, 6 of 10 (60%) quasi-experimental, and 1 of 2 (50%) true experimental designs reported significant improvements in personality following participation in an exercise program. These figures are indicative of a trend towards less observable effects as experimental rigor improves. A somewhat disconcerting observation from Table 5.1 is that a relatively large number of the experiments investigating the exercise and personality relationship were pre-experimental designs. You will recall that this design category provides us with the least amount of experimental control and hence the least amount of confidence concerning cause-effect relationships. The preponderance of pre-experimental designs may be related to the observation made earlier in the chapter that the majority of these studies were conducted in the 1960s and 1970s, at a time when experimental rigor was less of a concern. Although these pre-experimental designs must be viewed with some caution, there does remain some grounds for quiet optimism. When the pre-experimental studies are discounted, there remain 7 of 12 studies (58%) that report significant improvements in personality following exercise. In addition, three of four recent studies employing acceptable quasi-experimental designs report significant results (Buchman et al., 1991; J. Hogan, 1989; Jasnoski et al., 1988). In summary, in spite of some of the weaker early pre-experimental designs, there does appear reasonable support for the supposition that chronic exercise may impact positively on participant personality.

TABLE 5.1
Empirical Research Investigating the Exercise/Personality Relationship

Study	Design	Participants	Controls	Fitness Demonstrated?	Psychological Instruments	Outcome
Buccola and Stone (1975)	Quasi-Experimental	Male elderly adults	No	Yes	Cattell 16 PF	Improved
Buchman, Sallis, Criqui, Dimsdale, and Kaplan (1991)	Quasi-Experimental	Male and female college students	No	Yes	Bortner Short Rating Scale, State-Trait Anxiety Scale	Improved
Darden (1972)	Pre-Experimental	Male adult weight-lifters	No	No	Cattell 16 PF	No Change
De Geus, Lorenz, Van Doornen, and Orlebeke (1993)	Quasi-Experimental	Male adults	Yes	Yes	Dutch Personality Questionnaire	No Change
Folkins, Lynch, and Gardner (1972)	Quasi-Experimental	Male and female college students	Yes	Yes	Multiple Affect Adjective Checklist	Improved (females)
Gary and Gutherie (1972)	Experimental	Male adult alcoholics	Yes	Yes	Tennessee Self-Concept Scale	Improved
D.V. Harris (1966)	Pre-Experimental	Female college students	No	Yes	Edwards Personality Preference Scale	No Change
Hartung and Farge (1977)	Pre-Experimental	Male adult runners	No	Yes	Cattell 16 PF	Improved
J. Hogan (1989)	Quasi-Experimental	Male adults	No	Yes	Hogan Personality Inventory, MMPI	Improved
Ismail and Trachtman (1973)	Pre-Experimental	Male adults	No	No	Cattell 16 PF	Improved
Ismail and Young (1977)	Quasi-Experimental	Male adults	No	Yes	Cattell 16 PF, Eysenck Personality Inventory	No Change
Jasnoski and Holmes (1981)	Pre-Experimental	Female college students	No	Yes	Cattell 16 PF, Personality Survey	Improved
Jasnoski, Holmes, and Banks (1988)	Quasi-Experimental	Male and female college students	No	Yes	Cattell 16 PF, Zung's Self-Rating Depression Scale	Improved
Jones and Weinhouse (1979)	Pre-Experimental	Male and female adults	No	Yes	Cattell 16 PF	Improved

TABLE 5.1   (cont.)

Study	Design	Participants	Controls	Fitness Demonstrated?	Psychological Instruments	Outcome
Mayo (1975)	Experimental	Female children	Yes	Yes	Cattell Junior-Senior High School Questionnaire	No Change
Renfrew and Bolton (1979)	Pre-Experimental	Male adults	No	No	Cattell 16 PF	Improved
Sharp and Reilly (1975)	Pre-Experimental	Male college students	No	Yes	MMPI	Improved
Tillman (1965)	Quasi-Experimental	Male high school students	Yes	Yes	Cattell 16 PF, Kuder Preference Record	No Change
Werner and Gottheil (1966)	Quasi-Experimental	Male college students	Yes	No	Cattell 16 PF	No Change
Young and Ismail (1976)	Quasi-Experimental	Male adults	No	Yes	Cattell 16 PF, Eysenck Personality Inventory	Improved

Exercise and Personality: Suggested Mechanisms of Change

Because personality has been depicted as a complex of characteristics that distinguishes an individual, it becomes very difficult to isolate a specific mechanism (or mechanisms) with potential to explain the exercise and personality relationship. In contrast to the exercise and mood relationship (chapter 6), personality involves relatively enduring traits rather than the transient states characterized by mood. As such, the short-term explanations provided by the monoamine, endorphin, thermogenic, and distraction hypotheses appear to be of limited value in explaining the exercise and personality relationship. The only way the four exercise and mental health hypotheses could explain the exercise and personality relationship is if the exercise program is maintained, and the physiological and psychological changes are cumulative. At present, no empirical research has been located attempting to explain the exercise and personality relationship in terms of the monoamine, endorphin, thermogenic, or distraction hypotheses. An excellent review by Dienstbier (1984), however, hints at the possibility of such relationships' existing. In attempting to explain how exercise impacts on personality, Dienstibier suggests the following four possible mediators of personality change: (a) physiological changes, (b) perception of physical changes, (c) changes in patterns of socializing or living, and (d) changes in expectation. A brief explanation of each proposed mediator follows.

Physiological Changes

Dienstbier (1984) feels that physiological changes may impact on personality in two possible ways. First, regular exercise may result in a training effect. A training effect refers to physiological changes that result in increased capacity induced by constant use and is often accompanied by peripheral changes (e.g., increased muscle tone, increased muscle mass). Of importance to this discussion is a turn-of-the-century theory that emphasized the importance of feedback of peripheral changes in the experience of emotion. This viewpoint has gained renewed acceptance in the literature (Fehr & Stern, 1970). Part of the reason for the theory's resurgence is the observation that a variety of drugs whose effect is largely or exclusively peripheral affect emotional states (Dienstbier, 1979). In keeping with this theory, Dienstbier (1984) suggests that exercise, which causes peripheral changes, should influence the participant's emotional experience.

The second way Dienstbier feels exercise may influence personality physiologically is by its effect on brain chemistry. He believes the previously documented increases in endorphins and neural transmitters such as noradrenalin and acetylcholine following exercise may have long-term as well as short-term effects, resulting in a "training effect" in the brain. This suggests central nervous system physiological changes may impact directly on personality in a cumulative fashion. Dienstbier further speculates that the changes in balance between introversion and extroversion may be caused by the long-term impact of exercise on brain chemistry. This viewpoint remains conjecture at this point in time.

Perception of Physical Changes

Participation in an exercise program often results in changes, such as a reduction in body fat, redistribution of weight, increased energy levels, and a more youthful appearance. Most individuals value these physical developments because they are viewed positively by society at large. For this reason, Dienstbier (1984) believes exercise should lead to an improved body image (and concomitantly improved personality) in the following manner:

> One need not look deeply into the literature of personality and developmental psychology to determine that one of the most durable "truths" of those disciplines is that a positive body image contributes significantly to a generally positive self-concept, and that positive self-concept or high self-esteem correlates with general psychological health by almost any reasonable definition of that concept. (pp. 256-257)

Changes in Patterns of Socializing and Living

Morgan (1976) has suggested that runners often "get religion." In other words, an individual begins to realize that if exercise can bring about such substantial physical improvements, then changes in other such areas as patterns of drinking, eating, smoking, and sleeping may add to these benefits and make exercise easier and more successful. This viewpoint suggests a "domino effect" of exercise, in which exercise impacts on a variety of areas that ultimately influence our overall personality. Although untested, this viewpoint possesses a good degree of intuitive merit. Future research should more thoroughly investigate this hypothesis by collecting qualitative data on life-style changes associated with changes in exercise patterns.

Changes in Expectation

A final manner in which Dienstbier (1984) believes exercise may affect personality involves the participant's expectation. The tremendous popularization of exercise has resulted in a "knowledge explosion" of the positive benefits of regular exercise on mental health. According to Dienstbier, when the participant is convinced of the benefits, motivation to continue exercising remains high. In addition, the potential for a placebo effect is increased. In circumstances such as these, people may experience real improvements because of their expectations rather than because of the exercise program itself. This hypothesis aligns closely with the concept of self-efficacy/skills mastery discussed in chapter 4. By improving the participant's self-efficacy, the potential exists for exercise to make a small contribution to overall personality development.

Summary and Conclusions

The majority of studies investigating the exercise and personality relationship were conducted in the 1960s and 1970s. Since that time, very few empirical studies have been performed. This is probably reflective of the trend towards increased focus on psychological states rather than psychological traits. Participation in chronic exercise programs appears to be associated with improvements in personality, although the results remain somewhat inconsistent. In terms of specific personality dimensions, little consistency exists across the numerous studies. Only the subscale of "self-sufficient" appears to be frequently improved with prolonged involvement in an exercise program. Jogging appears to be the physical activity most often associated with positive changes in personality, although this observation must be viewed with caution, because so few other exercise modes have been employed. It is likely any aerobic physical activity will have the same beneficial results. Because personality represents relatively stable traits, longer exercise programs probably have a greater impact on participant personality than do shorter programs. Exercise appears to have a greater impact on personality when fitness gains are documented, although this may simply be related to the fact that an exercise program must be performed a relatively long period of time to improve participant fitness. The exact mechanism explaining the exercise and personality relationship has not been clearly established, although perceptions of physical change may be important.

Suggested Readings

Auweele, Y.V., De Cuyper, B., Van Mele, V., & Rzewnicki, R. (1993). Elite performance and personality: From description and prediction to diagnosis and intervention. In R. Singer, M. Murphy, & L. Tennant (Eds.), *Handbook of research on sport psychology* (pp. 257-289). New York: Macmillan.

Buchman, B.P., Sallis, J.F., Criqui, M.H., Dimsdale, J.E., & Kaplan, R.M. (1991). Physical activity, physical fitness, and psychological characteristics of medical students. *Journal of Psychosomatic Research, 35,* 197-208.

De Geus, E.J., VanDoornen, L.J., & Orlebeke, J.F. (1993). Regular exercise and aerobic fitness in relation to psychosocial make-up and physiological stress reactivity. *Psychosomatic Medicine, 55,* 347-363.

Hogan, J. (1989). Personality correlates of physical fitness. *Journal of Personality and Social Psychology, 56,* 284-288.

Jasnoski, M., Holmes, D.S., & Banks, D.L. (1988). Changes in personality associated with changes in aerobic and anaerobic fitness in women and men. *Journal of Psychosomatic Research, 32,* 273-276.

Morgan, W.P. (1980b). Sport personology: The credulous-skeptical argument in perspective. In W.F. Straub (Ed.), *Sport psychology: An analysis of athlete behavior* (2nd Ed.). Ithaca, NY: Mouvement Publications.

Rushall, B.S. (1973). The status of personality research and application in sports and physical education. *Journal of Sports Medicine and Physical Fitness, 13,* 281-290.

Chapter 6

EXERCISE AND MOOD

Our mood is affected in a variety of ways. A reprimand from our boss, a snub from a significant other, a flat tire, or the loss of a wallet are all capable of putting us into a bad mood. Similarly, a pat on the back, an enjoyable date, or a lottery ticket win can immediately put us back into an excellent frame of mind. It is normal to experience temporary mood swings. Most of us get the blues from time to time. Other days, we feel on top of the world, without always knowing why. These fluctuations in mood are natural and are part of everyday living. Only in the cases of bipolar affective disorder are these moodswings a cause for alarm (Fieve, 1989).

The objectives of this chapter are to (a) introduce the concept of mood, (b) briefly examine traditional treatments for problems with affect, (c) point out the potential of exercise for impacting positively on the participant's mood, (d) identify aspects of mood most often affected by exercise, (e) analyze and synthesize the empirical research to establish characteristics of exercise that lead to the best mood improvements, (f) provide exercise prescription guidelines for improving mood, and (g) suggest possible explanations concerning how exercise may impact on mood.

Defining Mood

The Webster Dictionary defines mood as "a conscious state of mind or predominant emotion." Mood may also be viewed as transient, fluctuating affective states. Recent research suggests mood may be further categorized as having both positive and negative affects. Positive affect reflects the individual's level of pleasurable engagement with the environment and is characterized by mental alertness, enthusiasm, energy, and determination. In contrast, negative affect reflects the person's general level of subjective distress, as witnessed by anger, guilt, fear, tension, sadness, scorn, and distrust (McIntyre, Watson, & Cunningham, 1990).

These states, or moods, are very situation specific. In contrast to the more basic personality traits, which suggest a predisposition to behave in a certain way regardless of the situation, mood states simply reflect how we feel at a particular moment in time. As such, they are far less predictive of how an individual will behave across a variety of situations. Nevertheless, the concept of mood is very important to most individuals. How we feel on a day-to-day basis is a primary concern as we go about our daily activities. It also determines, to a certain degree, our motivation and effectiveness in performing our everyday functions. It is probably for this reason that mood has been a psychological construct of major interest to the practitioner and layman alike.

Recognizing Mood Problems

Because mood involves such situation specific and transient psychological states, it is not always easy to recognize problems in mood that are of sufficient magnitude to require professional intervention. For this reason, chapter 6 will focus primarily on nonclinical mood problems. In other words, how do we recognize day-to-day mood problems in the general population? Two of the most frequently used methods involve behavioral observation and simple communication. If we are observant, it is not uncommon to notice individuals who are experiencing mood problems. These people may appear sad, nervous, angry, or even listless. In terms of communication, they frequently complain of feeling down, anxious, annoyed, or tired. In each of these cases, it is likely the person is suffering from some degree of negative mood state. In most cases, these fluctuations are within normal limits for the general population.

A somewhat more objective method of recognizing mood problems involves the use of psychometric instruments. The Profile of Mood States (McNair et al., 1971) was designed to meet the need for a rapid, economical method of identifying and assessing transient, fluctuating affective states. The instrument consists of 65 five-point adjective rating scales factored into the following six mood scores: (a) tension-anxiety, (b) depression-dejection, (c) anger-hostility, (d) vigor-activity, (e) fatigue-inertia, and (f) confusion-bewilderment (Eichman, 1978). The POMS was originally developed as a means of measuring "last week including today" kinds of mood states in individuals undergoing counseling or psychotherapy. This would probably explain why there is reduced emphasis on positive mood states in the POMS (only vigor-activity could be considered positive). Because the instrument was designed for use with psychiatric outpatients, its primary function was to identify mood improvements rather than degrees of positive mood states. Because of its sensitivity to mood improvements in a wide variety of settings, the POMS has been adapted almost exclusively into the exercise and mood literature. Intitially, Morgan (1981, 1982, 1985) pioneered the POMS use in sport to spot negative shifts in mood. Since that time, it has been employed frequently to ascertain mood changes with exercise.

Traditional Treatments for Mood Problems

For most individuals, problems with mood usually disappear on their own within a relatively short period of time. For others, these problems are more recurrent and require some form of intervention. In cases of this nature, trained professionals often must resort to psychotropic medication.

When mood problems are not of sufficient severity to require drug therapy, they often respond well to counseling by a trained professional. In these sessions, the client is encouraged to talk about his or her problems and seek solutions in consultation with the counselor. Cognitive therapy and cognitive behavior modification are among the most popular treatments for problems with mood. Cognitive therapy attempts to eliminate cognitive distortions that are causing the client to feel bad. An excellent example of this technique is provided in the book *Feeling Good: The New Mood Therapy* by Burns (1980). In addition, some success has been experienced by cognitive behavior modification, in which the client utilizes positive self-statements and imagery to improve his or her mood. A final activity that appears to have potential for improving mood is exercise. The remainder of the chapter will investigate this exercise and mood relationship.

The Exercise and Mood Relationship

It is tempting to speculate that interest in the relationship between exercise and mood states developed as a result of the frequently quoted "feel better" phenomenon reported after exercise. Those who involve themselves in physical exercise on a regular basis commonly report that exercising makes them feel good. This feel better phenomenon is frequently noted in the literature (Brunner, 1969; Burgess, 1976; D.V. Harris, 1978; Morgan, 1973, 1979c; Morgan et al., 1970; Morgan, Roberts, & Feinerman, 1971; W.T.

Roth, 1974; Sharkey, 1979). Although the feel better phenomenon appears to be pervasive in the exercise literature, this subjective feeling is not always supported by changes in objective test scores (Sachs, 1984b). Even so, this feeling of well-being after exercise appears to have played a significant role in promoting participation in physical activity. It has also served a heuristic function in terms of generating research investigating the exercise and mood relationship.

Elements of Mood Influenced by Exercise

Because mood is a multidimensional concept, it is not sufficient merely to report improvements or nonimprovements in mood following involvement in an exercise program. Although this technique has been utilized in several recent reviews (Doan & Scherman, 1987; Folkins & Sime, 1981; Gleser & Mendelberg, 1990; Leith & Taylor, 1990), a more appropriate analysis involves looking at the specific elements of mood affected by the exercise process. Utilization of a variety of psychometric instruments makes a review of this nature possible.

POMS measures of mood change following exercise. The majority of studies examining the exercise and mood association have employed the Profile of Mood States (McNair et al., 1971). An overview of studies employing the POMS reveals that exercise has been consistently associated with improvements in tension-anxiety (Berger & Owen, 1983, 1988, 1992; Berger, Owen, & Man, 1993; Blumenthal et al., 1982; Fremont & Craighead, 1987; Jin, 1989; Kowal et al., 1978; Lichtman & Poster, 1983; Maroulakis & Zervas, 1993; McGowan, Pierce, & Jordan, 1991; Moses, Steptoe, Mathews, & Edwards, 1989; D.L. Roth, 1989; Shephard, Kavanaugh, & Klavora, 1985; C.W. Simons & Birkimer, 1988; Steptoe, Edwards, Moses, & Mathews, 1989; Steptoe et al., 1993; R. Weinberg, Jackson, & Kolodny, 1988; Wilfley & Kunce, 1986; Zorn, 1989), depression-dejection (Berger & Owen, 1983, 1988; Berger et al., 1993; Blumenthal et al., 1982; Dyer & Crouch, 1987, 1988; Fremont & Craighead, 1987; Kowal et al., 1978; Lichtman & Poster, 1983; Maroulakis & Zervas, 1993; Shephard et al., 1985; Steptoe et al., 1989, 1993; R. Weinberg et al., 1988; V.E. Wilson, Morley, & Bird, 1980; Zorn, 1989), anger-hostility (Berger & Owen, 1983, 1988; Berger et al., 1993; Dyer & Crouch, 1987; Fremont & Craighead, 1987; Jin, 1989; Lichtman & Poster, 1983; Maroulakis & Zervas, 1993; Shephard et al., 1985; C.W. Simons & Birkimer, 1988; R. Weinberg et al.,

1988; V.E. Wilson et al., 1980), vigor-activity (Berger & Owen, 1983; Berger et al., 1993; Blumenthal et al., 1982; Dyer & Crouch, 1988; Flory & Holmes, 1991; Jin, 1989; Kowal et al., 1978; Maroulakis & Zervas, 1993; Shephard et al., 1985; Steptoe et al., 1989; V.E. Wilson et al., 1980), fatigue-inertia (Berger & Owen, 1988; Blumenthal et al., 1982; Fremont & Craighead, 1987; Jin, 1989; Kowal et al., 1978; Lichtman & Poster, 1983; Shephard et al., 1985; Steptoe et al., 1989; R. Weinberg et al., 1988), and confusion-bewilderment (Berger & Owen, 1983, 1988; Berger et al., 1993; Dyer & Crouch, 1987, 1988; Fremont & Craighead, 1987; Jin, 1989; Kowal et al., 1978; Maroulakis & Zervas, 1993; McGowan et al., 1991; Moses et al., 1989; Roth, 1989; Shephard et al., 1985; C.W. Simons & Birkimer, 1988; Steptoe et al., 1993; R. Weinberg et al., 1988; V.E. Wilson et al., 1980).

Prescription Guideline 6.1
    A substantial body of research reveals exercise to be associated with participant mood improvements in tension-anxiety, depression-dejection, anger-hostility, vigor-activity, fatigue-inertia, and confusion-bewilderment. Anxiety, depression, and confusion are the three subscales most frequently showing improvement.

Surprisingly, only four studies utilizing the POMS reported no changes in any of the six mood variables (Frazier & Nagy, 1989; J.R. Hughes, Casal, & Leon, 1986; McGowan et al., 1993; Williams & Getty, 1986). These findings, taken in conjunction, suggest that the Profile of Mood States is a psychometric instrument very sensitive to mood changes associated with exercise and that exercise is associated with improvements in several aspects of mood in the majority of studies. A notable exception to this viewpoint concerns the research (Morgan et al., 1987; Morgan et al., 1988) on over-training in elite athletes. In these studies, overtraining was found to be associated with worsened mood scores. This concept will be more fully explored in chapter 8. The suggestion by D.R. Brown (1992) that the POMS may not be appropriate for exercise and mood due to a "floor effect," or positive initial mood scores, does not appear warranted on the basis of previously cited research.

Other measures of mood change following exercise. Although the POMS has been used almost exclusively in the exercise and mood literature, recent research has started to employ psychometric instruments that differentiate between positive and negative aspects of mood. The Mood Adjective Check-list (Nowlis, 1965) is a 33-adjective checklist that measures positive and negative mood states. The seven factors constituting these mood states include sadness, anxiety, aggression, fatigue, surgency, vigor, and elation. The first four factors represent negative affects, whereas the last three represent positive affects. A study by Lennox, Bedell, and Stone (1990) utilized the Mood Adjective Checklist to measure the effect of aerobic (walking/jogging) and anaerobic exercise (weight lifting/volleyball) on participant mood states. At the conclusion of a 13-week program, no changes in any of the mood subscales were observed. Similar findings were reported by Gauvin (1989) on a sample of 122 male and female adults ranging from 18 to 77 years of age. Gauvin employed a psychometric instrument known as the Affectometer (Kamman & Flett, 1983). This paper and pencil questionnaire measures the frequency of positive and negative affect. Two subscales are available that require the subjects to rate on a 5-point scale the frequency with which they experience feelings described by two series of 20 statements or adjectives. Each scale yields two scores, which range from 5 to 50, reflecting the frequency of positive and negative affect. This instrument was administered to four experimental groups representing autonomous exercisers, fitness program enrollees, fitness program drop-outs, and nonexercisers. Results of the study revealed no significant differences between the groups in terms of frequency of positive or negative affect. It is important to note, however, that this study was cross-sectional, comparing the groups at one specific point in time. It would be valuable for future research to employ a longitudinal design, comparing exercisers and nonexercisers in terms of the effects of exercise on positive and negative affect over time. In a study of this nature, exercise may be found to significantly increase positive affect and decrease negative affect in a cumulative fashion. Within group comparisons over time are needed to test this hypothesis.

Partial support for this position is provided by McIntyre et al. (1990). In this study, a relatively new instrument called the Positive Affect and Negative Affect Schedule (PANAS), developed by Watson, Clark, and Tellegen (1988) was utilized. The PANAS contains 10-item positive affect and negative affect scales. The positive affect scale consists of the mood descriptors active, alert, attentive, determined, enthusiastic, excited, inspired, interested, proud, and strong. The negative affect scale consists of the descriptors afraid, ashamed, distressed, guilty, hostile, irritable, jittery, nervous, scared, and upset. The subjects rated the extent to which they were experiencing each mood descriptor at that moment. The ratings were performed on a 5-point scale. Eighteen male and female undergraduate students completed a PANAS at the beginning of a 1-week period to establish baseline levels of positive and negative affect. They were then administered three additional PANAS within the week. One was performed after social interaction, one after exercise, and another prior to a stressful test. The resulting scores obtained after each of these conditions were then compared to original baseline scores. Statistical comparisons revealed that both exercise and social interaction significantly increased positive affect, but exerted no influence on negative affect.

Types of Exercise Associated With Changes in Mood

The majority of studies investigating the exercise and mood relationship utilized running and/or walking as the mode of physical activity(Blumenthal et al., 1982; Dyer & Crouch, 1987, 1988; Folkins, 1976; Fremont & Craighead, 1987; Shephard et al., 1985; C.W. Simons & Birkimer, 1988; Steptoe et al., 1993; Wilfley & Kunce, 1986; V.E. Wilson et al., 1980). However, a variety of other types of exercise that have been associated with improvements in mood include swimming (Berger & Owen, 1983, 1992; Berger et al., 1993), cycling (Hardy & Rejeski, 1989; D.L. Roth, 1989), yoga (Berger & Owen, 1988), tai chi (Jin, 1989), basic training in an army camp (Kowal et al., 1978), rowing (Douchamps-Riboux, Heinz, & Douchamps, 1989), weight lifting (McGowan et al., 1991; Norvell & Belles, 1993), aerobic dance (Flory & Holmes, 1991; Maroulakis & Zervas, 1993), as well as "unspecified" exercise programs (Frazier & Nagy, 1989; Gauvin, 1989; Zorn, 1989).

Prescription Guideline 6.2
   The most frequent and consistent mood improvements following exercise have been associated with jogging and/or walking programs. Although a variety of other physical activities have resulted in mood improvements, the majority of exercise modes have been aerobic.

Comparing exercise types. Several researchers have attempted to determine if certain exercise modes are superior to others in terms of their potential to impact on mood. A study by Berger and Owen (1988) compared the effects of swimming, body conditioning, hatha yoga, and fencing on mood states in a sample of 170 male and female college undergraduates. All exercises were performed 2 days per week, 40 minutes per session, for 14 weeks. Exercise intensity was considered to be moderate because all activities were performed at the beginner level, although this factor was not controlled across exercise types. Mood changes were measured by means of the POMS on three separate occasions. These mood scores were then averaged across the

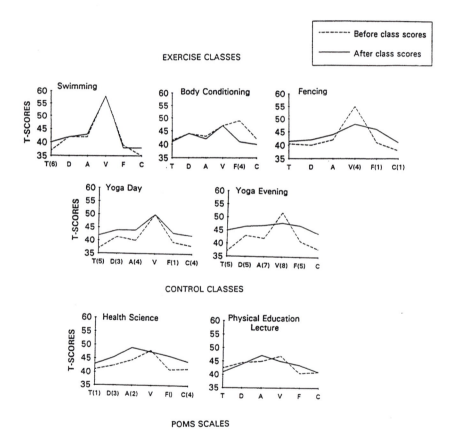

Figure 6.1. Mean POMS t scores averaged across 3 days comparing 4 different types of exercise with 2 classroom control conditions. The POMS subscales include Tension (T), Depression (D), Anger (A), Vigor (V), Fatigue (F), and Confusion (C).

Note. From "Stress reduction and mood enhancement in four exercise modes: Swimming, body conditioning, hatha yoga, and fencing" by B.G. Berger and D.R. Owen, 1988, *Research Quarterly for Exercise and Sport, 59*, p.153. Copyright © 1988 by the American Alliance for Health, Physical Education, Recreation, and Dance. Reprinted by permission.

three testing sessions. Results of the study are portrayed in Figure 6.1. Participants in yoga reported significant improvements in anxiety, depression, anger, fatigue, and confusion after class on all three occasions. The fencing group reported improvements only in the vigor dimension, whereas the body-conditioning group experienced a significant improvement in fatigue, but no other mood changes. The swimming group demonstrated significantly less anxiety and confusion after swimming, but this change was observed only on the first day of testing. These findings did not support the original hypothesis that the swimming group would demonstrate the greatest improvements in mood because it involved the greatest aerobic involvement. The authors noted, however, that the swimmers had unusually positive initial mood scores prior to the exercise sessions and that these elevated mood scores left little room for improvements following swimming. A future study should attempt to replicate this experiment with the notable exception of matching subjects in each exercise group by initial mood scores. By making this experimental design adjustment, it is likely that the swimming condition would compare more favorably to the other exercise modes. A study of this nature would also enable the researcher to establish a more meaningful ranking of exercises most conducive to mood changes.

A study by Dyer and Crouch (1988) has also attempted to compare different types of exercise in terms of their mood change potential. Seventy male and female college undergraduates were recruited from classes in jogging/conditioning, weight training, aerobic dance, and a control group from introductory psychology. A time-series design was employed in which all participants completed eight POMS questionnaires, four during the second week of classes, then four at midsemester (approximately 6 weeks later). Results of this experiment are shown in Figure 6.2. The authors reported that runners had a significantly more positive mood profile than did nonexercisers and a somewhat more positive one than did weightlifters. The mood profiles of runners and aerobic dancers were similar. Dyer and Crouch concluded that changes in moods across time in relation to activity and across semester suggest that exercise (especially aerobic exercise) helps the participant cope with stress and have a more positive mood profile.

Prescription Guideline 6.3

Research comparing exercise modes has been unable to identify one type of physical activity as being superior to another. It, therefore, appears any form of exercise has potential to impact positively on participant mood. This makes exercise selection a personal choice.

It is important that future studies begin to examine qualitative aspects of exercise and their relationship to mood, rather than merely to compare isolated exercises. For example, what are the differential effects of (a) aerobic vs. nonaerobic exercise, (b) social vs. autonomous participation, (c) competitive vs. noncompetitive activities, and (d) rhythmical vs. nonrhythmical exercise on participant mood states? Another important research question is to determine if the effects of different exercise types have differential effects on certain mood states. It seems reasonable to hypothesize that aerobic, social, rhythmical, and noncompetitive exercise would result in the greatest mood improvements for the majority of participants. To date, these relationships have not been thoroughly tested.

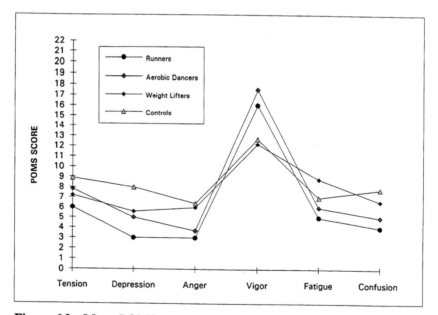

Figure 6.2. Mean POMS scores at 3 hr before activity and 10 min after activity for runners (n=17), aerobic dancers (n=17), weight lifters (n=18), and controls (n=18). Arrows show direction of change, with each arrow's point of origin denoting 3 hr before activity and its end 10 min after.

Note. From "Effects of running and other activities on moods" by J.B. Dyer and J.G. Crouch, 1988, *Perceptual and Motor Skills, 67,* p.47. Copyright © 1988 by *Perceptual and Motor Skills.* Reprinted by permission.

Length of exercise program. Significant improvements in mood have been found following exercise programs lasting ≥ 5 months (Dyer & Crouch, 1987; Gauvin, 1989; Jin, 1989; Shephard et al., 1985; V.E. Wilson et al., 1980), 12-15 weeks (Berger & Owen, 1983, 1988, 1992; Berger et al., 1993; Dyer & Crouch, 1988; Folkins, 1976; Frazier & Nagy, 1989; J.R. Hughes et al., 1986; Lennox et al., 1990), and 6-10 weeks (Blumenthal et al., 1982; Fremont & Craighead, 1987; Kowal et al., 1978; Moses et al., 1989; C.W. Simons & Birkimer, 1988; Steptoe et al., 1989, 1993; Wilfley & Kunce, 1986; Williams & Getty, 1986).

> **Prescription Guideline 6.4**
> **Exercise programs ranging from 6 weeks to over 5 months have produced significant improvements in participants' mood scores. The exact length of the exercise program does not appear critical for improvements in mood to be experienced.**

This viewpoint is further reinforced by the increasing number of recent studies reporting mood improvements after a single bout of exercise (Douchamps-Riboux et al., 1989; Flory & Holmes, 1991; Hardy & Rejeski, 1989; Maroulakis & Zervas, 1993; McGowan et al., 1991; McIntyre et al., 1990; D.L. Roth, 1989; R. Weinberg et al., 1988).

> **Prescription Guideline 6.5**
> **Significant improvements in participant mood scores have been reported after single bouts of exercise. These changes are likely more transient than those occurring with chronic participation in exercise.**

An experiment by McGowan et al. (1991), for example, compared 65-75 minutes of running, weight-lifting, and karate on mood changes in 72 male and female college students. POMS scores obtained after these single bouts of activity revealed that both running and weight-lifting groups experienced significant reductions in the tension and confusion subscales of mood. No changes were seen in the karate group. This study suggests that even a single bout of exercise has the potential to produce positive changes in affect. Identifying these acute changes in the POMS has been made possible since the instructional set of the instrument was altered to include "right now" aspects of mood. This finding is consistent with the "feel better" phenomenon discussed earlier. An important question that must be addressed by future research pertains to how long these positive effects last. Not one study investigating the effect of a single bout of exercise on mood has employed a follow-up measure. It would be valuable for a future experiment to conduct follow-up measures at specified intervals (e.g., 1, 2, 3,...hr.) following completion of the activity. Research of this nature will help us determine how long the effects of exercise on mood last. A logical extension of this research will help us determine how often we must exercise to maintain these positive benefits on mood. To answer this question, future research will also have to perform follow-up measures at longer intervals after the exercise session (e.g., 1, 2, and 3 days). If it could be ascertained that the positive mood changes following exercise last for 2 days, for example, an individual would only have to exercise an average of 3 1/2 times per week to maintain mood benefits. It seems reasonable to assume that the positive affect associated with exercise will be determined to last at least several hours after completion of the activity. To date, this hypothesis remains untested.

Exercise frequency. The majority of studies reviewed required exercise to be performed three times per week (Blumenthal et al., 1982; Dyer & Crouch, 1987, 1988; Folkins, 1976; Fremont & Craighead, 1987; Norvell &: Belles, 1993; Wilfley & Kunce, 1986). Exercise frequencies of one time per week (Berger & Owen, 1988; R. Weinberg et al., 1988), two times per week (Berger & Owen, 1983, 1992; Berger et al., 1993; C.W. Simons & Birkimer, 1988), four times per week (Steptoe et al., 1993); and seven times per week (Kowal et al, 1978; V.E. Wilson et al., 1980) have also been associated with improved mood in the participants.

> **Prescription Guideline 6.6**
> To experience consistent positive mood changes, exercise should be performed a minimum of three or four times per week. Although mood improvements have been reported with greater exercise frequencies, this approach has also resulted in worsened affect in some cases.

A study by J.R. Hughes et al. (1986) required a sample of male adults to exercise five times per week either walking a treadmill for 45 minutes or stairclimbing 10 flights of stairs for a comparable period of time. At the conclusion of a 12-week exercise program, no changes in any of the POMS subscales were reported. Although it is tempting to suggest that exercising five times per week may be too often (and thereby too taxing) to experience mood improvements, a more likely explanation involves the actual nature of exercise in this study. Both exercise conditions could be considered repetitive and boring. They are both conducted indoors in the absence of stimulation. It, therefore, seems reasonable to suggest that the failure of this study to report improvements in mood is not related to an increased frequency of exercise sessions. This view is further supported by the Kowal et al. (1978) and V.E. Wilson et al. (1980) studies, both reporting mood improvements with exercise frequencies of seven times per week. This question may ultimately be answered by a future study that employs a particular type of exercise, then manipulates experimental treatments employing different frequencies of this exercise. Research of this nature will likely establish an optimal frequency (3 or 4 times per week) for improving mood in the participants.

Exercise intensity. Many of the studies examining the exercise and mood relationship do not report exercise intensities. Of those that do, exercise intensities of 60%-85% maximum heart rates or VO2 max. were utilized. Because the majority of these studies report exercise intensities within a particular range, such as 70%-85% (Blumenthal et al., 1982; Folkins, 1976), 65%-85% (Frazier & Nagy, 1989), and 60%-80% (Flory & Holmes, 1991; Maroulakis & Zervas, 1993; Steptoe et al., 1993) maximum heart rates, it becomes impossible to compare exercise intensities in terms of their mood-elevating effects. A study by Hardy and Rejeski (1989) attempted to address this issue. A sample of 30 male college students enrolled in physical activity courses took part in the experiment. The experimental trial consisted of all subjects cycling at 30%, 60%, and 90% of their maximum aerobic power (VO2 max.). Feeling states in the subjects were ascertained by means of the Feeling Scale (FS) developed by Rejeski, Best, Griffith, and Kenney (1987). The feeling scale is presented in an 11-point bipolar good/bad format, ranging from +5 to -5. Verbal anchors are provided at the 0 point, and all odd integers (+5 = very good, +3 = good, +1 = fairly good, 0 = neutral, -1 = fairly bad, -3 = bad, and -5 = very bad). The perceived intensity of the exercise was measured by the Rating of Perceived Exertion (RPE) scale, developed by Borg (1985). Near the completion of each 4-minute bout of exercise, RPEs and FS ratings were measured. The results of this study revealed that increases in exercise intensity yielded higher RPES and more negative feeling states, suggesting that ratings of perceived exertion are moderately correlated with feeling states. This finding suggests that as exercise becomes more strenuous, mood appears to worsen, although this effect is likely transitory. This observation led Hardy and Rejeski (1989) to recommend that future research should begin to explore the connection between feeling states and the mental health consequences of exercise, with the former possibly being a prerequisite to the latter. In other words, only exercise that makes us feel good may be good for our mental health.

Prescription Guidline 6.7

Moderate-intensity exercise appears to have the best potential to impact on participant mood states. Although high-intensity exercise has also been associated with significant improvements, it has also produced negative results in some instances. In addition, moderate-intensity physical activity is safer and more enjoyable for most individuals.

It is important that future research take this a step further by attempting to establish how the exercise makes us feel good. The development of a short-form of meaningful affective adjectives and the utilization of a format similar to the Feeling Scale would provide valuable information in terms of those elements of mood impacted by different exercise intensities. Another suggestion for future research would be to utilize instruments such as the PANAS (Watson et al., 1988) or the Affectometer (Kamman & Flett, 1983) to ascertain the effect of different exercise intensities on positive versus negative affect. Research conducted to date (Hardy & Rejeski, 1989) suggests that higher exercise intensities may be associated with higher negative affect, whereas low to moderate intensities may produce increased positive affect. Research is needed to test this hypothesis.

Only one other study (Moses et al., 1989) was located that attempted to establish the relationship between different exercise intensities and changes in mood. The subjects for this experiment were 75 sedentary male and female adults. The subjects were randomly assigned to one of four experimental treatments. A high-exercise group engaged in a walk/jog program four times per week for 15-60 minutes at 70%-75% maximum heart rate. A moderate-exercise group also participated in walking/jogging activity four times per week for 20 minutes at 60% maximum heart rate. An attention-placebo group was involved with strength, mobility, and flexibility training four times per week for 30 minutes at 50% maximum heart rate. A fourth group served as waiting-list control. Results of this study revealed that only the high-exercise group experienced improvements in fitness. However, only the moderate-exercise group demonstrated significant mood improvements in the POMS tension-anxiety subscale. The improvements were still manifest at the 3-month follow-up. These results are shown in Figure 6.3 (please note the log transformations used in the figure act to overaccentuate the degree of mood change). The authors interpreted these findings to sug-

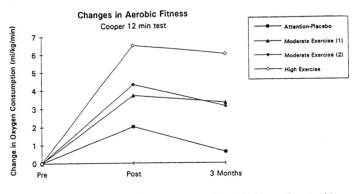

a)   Mean change in estimated maximum oxygen consumption calculated from performance of the 12 minute test pre- and post-training and at 3 month follow-up.

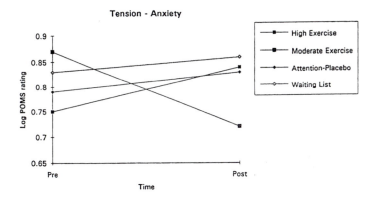

b)   Mean log transformed tension-anxiety score on the POMS for the four experimental conditions before and after training.

Figure 6.3. The relationship between aerobic fitness and mood change.
Note. **From "The effects of exercise training on mental well-being in the normal population: A controlled trial" by J. Moses, A. Steptoe, A. Mathews, & S. Edwards, 1989, *Journal of Psychosomatic Research, 33*, pp. 55-56. Copyright © 1989 by Pergamon Press. Reprinted by permission.**

gest that high-intensity exercise may be too demanding to improve psychological functioning. This viewpoint collaborates the findings of Hardy and Rejeski (1989) and points out the importance of further examination of the exercise intensity and mood change relationship.

Exercise duration. Most of the studies reviewed involved exercise sessions of 20 or more minutes, with the majority of studies falling in the 40- to 60-minute range (Berger & Owen, 1983, 1988; Berger et al., 1993; Blumenthal et al., 1982; Dyer & Crouch, 1987, 1988; Folkins, 1976; Wilfley & Kunce, 1986; Williams & Getty, 1986).

Prescription Guideline 6.8

A minimum of 20-minute exercise durations is recommended for improving participant mood. Although longer durations are cited in the literature, no evidence exists suggesting longer sessions are associated with more mood improvement.

No trends were observed in terms of exercise duration and mood changes in the participants. Not a single study was found comparing different durations in terms of their mood-enhancing effects. It would be valuable for future research to experimentally manipulate exercise durations, utilizing the same exercise mode, to determine the minimum exercise duration required to produce positive mood changes. This same question could be addressed by means of a single subject repeated measures design, in which mood measures are taken at prescribed intervals within a single bout of exercise as was done in the Hardy and Rejeski (1989) study. In the Hardy and Rejeski study, however, exercise intensity was the dependent variable rather than exercise duration. By maintaining the same exercise intensity, and taking dependent measures of mood at different durations (e.g., 5, 10, 15, 20...minutes), it will be possible to determine how long we must exercise to experience beneficial results. A study of this nature will also allow us to ascertain whether or not the effects of exercise on mood are cumulative. In other words, do the mood changes associated with exercise occur within the first 5 or 10 minutes and then plateau for the duration of the physical activity, or do the mood changes progress in increments throughout the entire session? Another possibility may be that undesirable mood changes take place as the exercise occurs, then are followed by a positive shift immediately following cessation of the exercise. Although mood improvements have been reported following exercise sessions of 20 minutes (Flory &

Holmes, 1991; Fremont & Craighead, 1987; McIntyre et al., 1990; Moses et al, 1989; D.L. Roth, 1989; Steptoe et al., 1989), no data are available utilizing shorter exercise durations. Previously cited research with state anxiety suggests future research will determine even short exercise durations to be associated with mood improvements in the participant.

Importance of Fitness Gains

To examine the effect of chronic participation in exercise programs on the more stable aspects mood, it is worthwhile to determine if fitness improvements are necessary for a positive psychological outcome. The majority of studies examining the exercise and mood relationship do not measure or report fitness changes in the participant. Of those studies that do document fitness gains, significant improvements in mood have been reported (Blumenthal et al., 1982; Folkins, 1976; Moses et al., 1989; Norvell & Belles, 1993; Shephard et al., 1985; C.W. Simons & Birkimer, 1988; Steptoe et al., 1989, 1993; Wilfley & Kunce, 1986), although three studies reporting improved fitness revealed no changes in participant mood (J.R. Hughes et al., 1986; Lennox et al., 1990; Williams & Getty, 1986). An even larger number of studies not documenting fitness gains have also been associated with mood improvements (Berger & Owen, 1983, 1988, 1992; Berger et al., 1993; Dyer & Crouch, 1987, 1988; Flory & Holmes, 1991; Fremont & Craighead, 1987; Jin, 1989; Lichtman & Poster, 1983; McGowan et al., 1991; McIntyre et al., 1990; R. Weinberg et al., 1988; V.E. Wilson et al., 1980; Zorn, 1989).

> **Prescription Guideline 6.9**
> Taken cumulatively, research findings suggest improvements in fitness are not necessary for the participant to experience beneficial mood effects following exercise. As an important caveat, fitness changes were invariably measured in terms of aerobic power. No research is available that attempts to link body composition, muscular strength/endurance, or flexibility fitness measures to postexercise mood states.

These findings suggest improvements in fitness are not necessary in order for the participant to experience beneficial mood effects following exercise. A study by Steptoe et al. (1989) provides statistical support for this viewpoint. The authors examined the effects of a moderate aerobic training program (ATP) and an attention-placebo strength and flexibility training program (APP) on the mood of 33 clinically anxious adults aged 20 through 60 years. The ATP group exercised four times per week for 20 minutes at 60%-65% maximum heart rate. The APP group also exercised four times per week for 20 minutes at 50% maximum heart rate. At the conclusion of the 10 week program, only the ATP group demonstrated significant POMS reductions in tension and depression. These effects were maintained at the 3-month follow-up session. When product moment correlations were calculated between changes in aerobic fitness and psychological responses, no significant correlations were observed. The authors thus concluded that changes in fitness are not a necessary prerequisite for mood improvements following exercise. They further suggest that psychological benefits accrue from psycho-physiological responses to stress following individual bouts of exercise and that these effects may accumulate over time independent of fitness changes. No empirical evidence for this viewpoint is presented in the study.

Population Trends

An overview of completed research reveals some variety in terms of sample populations chosen for experimentation. Healthy, asymptomatic subjects have been studied in the form of college students (Berger & Owen, 1983, 1988, 1992; Berger et al., 1993; Dyer & Crouch, 1988; Flory & Holmes, 1991; Hardy & Rejeski, 1989; McGowan et al., 1991; McIntyre et al., 1990; D.L. Roth, 1989; Shephard et al., 1985; R. Weinberg et al., 1988), and adults (Blumenthal et al., 1982; Douchamps-Riboux et al., 1989; Dyer & Crouch, 1987; Folkins, 1976; Frazier & Nagy, 1989; Gauvin, 1989; J.R. Hughes et al., 1986; Jin, 1989; Kowal et al., 1978; Lennox et al., 1990; Lichtman & Poster, 1983; Maroulakis & Zervas, 1993; McGowan et al., 1993; Moses et al., 1989; Norvell & Belles, 1993; C.W. Simons & Birkimer, 1988; Steptoe et al., 1993; Wilfley & Kunce, 1986; V.E. Wilson et al., 1980). In addition, special populations including depressed adults (Fremont & Craighead, 1987), anxious adults (Steptoe et al., 1989), cardiac patients (Shephard et al., 1985), and pregnant females (Williams & Getty, 1986; Zorn, 1989) were studied.

In summary, the majority of studies examining the exercise and mood relationship have utilized either healthy adults or college students as subjects. In most instances, these experiments have reported significant mood improvements following exercise. The small number of studies utilizing special populations and clinically symptomatic subjects does not allow for meaningful conclusions to be drawn on these samples. The research that has been conducted to date, however, appears promising. Fremont and Craighead (1987), for example, randomly assigned 61 subjects who had been classified as either mildly or moderately depressed to one of three experimental conditions: running only, cognitive therapy only, or combined running and cognitive therapy. At the conclusion of the 10 week program, all three groups experienced significant improvements in depression, confusion, anxiety, anger, and fatigue. No significant differences were found between the experimental conditions. The authors concluded that supervised involvement in aerobic exercise may be a cost-effective alternative treatment to traditional verbal therapy for mood disorders. A similar study by Steptoe et al. (1989) randomly assigned 33 clinically anxious male and female adults to either a moderate exercise group or an attention-placebo control. At the conclusion of the 10-week program, the exercise group who had exercised four times per week for 20 minutes a session reported significant improvements in tension-anxiety, confusion-bewilderment, and depression-dejection as measured by the POMS. These changes remained at a 3-month follow-up. The Fremont and Craighead (1987) and Steptoe et al. (1989) studies suggest that exercise has valuable potential for improving mood in patients who are clinically symptomatic in terms of depression and anxiety. The small number of studies, however, points out the need for replication studies on similar samples.

Quality of Completed Research -- Design Considerations

Now that an analysis and synthesis of available experiments have been performed, it is important to consider the quality of research that has investigated the exercise and mood relationship. This will be done by examining the experimental designs and comparing the results as research becomes more rigorously controlled. As a reference point, Table 6.1 summarizes completed research by design characteristics.

Thirty-four studies are summarized in Table 6.1. If we look at overall results, 26 of the 34 studies (77%) reported significant improvements in some aspect of mood following exercise. When we examine improvements by design category, 2 of 2 (100%) pre-experimental, 19 of 24 (79%) quasi-experimental, and 5 of 8 (63%) true experimental designs reported significant improvements. These figures are somewhat indicative of a trend towards less consistent findings as experimental rigor improves. This obser-

TABLE 6.1
Empirical Research Investigating the Exercise/Mood Relationship

Study	Design	Participants	Controls	Fitness Demonstrated?	Psychological Instruments	Outcome
Berger and Owen (1983)	Quasi-Experimental	Male and female college students	Yes	No	Profile of Mood States	Improved
Berger and Owen (1988)	Quasi-Experimental	Male and female college students	Yes	No	Profile of Mood States, State-Trait Anxiety Inventory	Improved
Berger and Owen (1992)	Experimental	Male and female college students	Yes	No	Profile of Mood States	Improved
Berger, Owen, and Man (1993)	Quasi-Experimental	Female college students	Yes	No	Profile of Mood States	Improved
Blumenthal, Williams, Needels, and Wallace (1982)	Quasi-Experimental	Male and female adults	Yes	Yes	Profile of Mood States, State-Trait Anxiety Inventory	Improved
Douchamps-Riboux, Heinz, and Douchamps (1989).	Quasi-Experimental	Male adult rowers	No	No	Unnamed Instrument	Worsened
Dyer and Crouch (1987)	Quasi-Experimental	Male and female adults	Yes	No	Profile of Mood States	Improved
Dyer and Crouch (1988)	Quasi-Experimental	Male and female college students	Yes	No	Profile of Mood States	Improved
Flory and Holmes (1991)	Quasi-Experimental	Female college students	Yes	No	Multiple Affect Adjective Checklist	Improved
Folkins (1976)	Quasi-experimental	Male adults	Yes	Yes	Multiple Affect Adjective Checklist	Improved
Frazier and Nagy (1989)	Quasi-Experimental	Female adult exercisers	No	No	Profile of Mood States	No Change
Fremont (1984)	Experimental	Male and female depressed adults	Yes	No	Unnamed Instruments	Improved
Fremont and Craighead (1987)	Quasi-Experimental	Male and female adults	No	No	Profile of Mood States, State-Trait Anxiety Inventory, Beck Depression Inventory	Improved
Hardy and Rejeski (1989)	Quasi-Experimental	Male college students	No	Yes	Multiple Affect Adjective Checklist	Worsened

TABLE 6.1   (Cont.)

Study	Design	Participants	Controls	Fitness Demonstrated	Psychological Instruments	Outcome
J.R. Hughes, Casal, and Leon (1986)	Experimental	Male adults	Yes	Yes	Profile of Mood States	No Change
Jin (1989)	Quasi-Experimental	Male and female tai chi members	No	No	Profile of Mood States	Improved
Kowal, Payton, and Vogel (1978)	Pre-Experimental	Male and female adults	No	Yes	Profile of Mood States, Eysenck Personality Inventory	Improved (males)
Lennox (1989)	Experimental	Male and female adults	Yes	Yes	Mood Adjective Checklist, Beck Depression Inventory	No Change
Lennox, Bedell, and Stone (1990)	Experimental	Male and female adults	Yes	Yes	Multiple Affect Adjective Checklist	No Change
Lichtman and Poster (1983)	Quasi-Experimental	Male and female adults	Yes	No	Profile of Mood States, Nowlis Mood Scale	Improved
Maroulakis and Zervas (1993)	Quasi-Experimental	Female adults	Yes	No	Profile of Mood States	Improved
McGowan, Pierce, Eastman, Tripathi, Dewey, and Olson (1993)	Quasi-Experimental	Male and female adults	No	No	Profile of Mood States	No Change
McIntyre, Watson, and Cunningham (1990)	Quasi-Experimental	Male and female college students	No	No	Positive Affect and Negative Affect Schedule	Improved
Norvell and Belles (1993)	Experimental	Male adults	Yes	Yes	Hopkins Symptoms Checklist	Improved
D.L. Roth (1989)	Experimental	Male and female college students	Yes	Yes	Profile of Mood States	Improved
Shephard, Kavanaugh, and Klavora (1985)	Quasi-Experimental	Male adult cardiac patients, male and female college students	Yes	Yes	Profile of Mood States	Improved
C.W. Simons and Birkimer (1988)	Quasi-Experimental	Male and female adults	Yes	Yes	Profile of Mood States	Improved
Steptoe, Edwards, Moses, and Mathews (1989)	Quasi-Experimental	Male and female anxious adults	No	Yes	Profile of Mood States	Improved

TABLE 6.1   (Cont.)

Study	Design	Participants	Controls	Fitness Demonstrated	Psychological Instruments	Outcome
Steptoe, Moses, Edwards, and Mathews (1993)	Experimental	Male and female sedentary anxious adults	Yes	Yes	Profile of Mood States	Improved
R. Weinberg, Jackson, and Kolodny (1988)	Quasi-Experimental	Male and female college students	Yes	No	Profile of Mood States, State-Trait Anxiety Inventory, Thayer's Adjective Checklist	Improved
Wilfley and Kunce (1986)	Quasi-Experimental	Male and female adults	No	Yes	Profile of Mood States, Tennessee Self-Concept Scale	Improved
Williams and Getty (1986)	Quasi-Experimental	Female adults (pregnant and not pregnant)	Yes	Yes	Profile of Mood States, Zung's Self-Rating Depression Scale	No Change
V.E. Wilson, Morley, and Bird (1980)	Pre-Experimental	Male adults	Yes	No	Profile of Mood States	Improved
Zorn (1989)	Quasi-Experimental	Female adults (pregnant and postpartum)	Yes	No	Profile of Mood States	Improved

vation must be tempered somewhat by the observation that only eight true experimental designs were performed. Such a small number makes it difficult to make meaningful generalizations. In addition, the fact that 79% of the quasi-experimental studies reported significant findings provides grounds for optimism. In summary, because only two of the experiments involved the relatively weak pre-experimental design category, it appears safe to suggest the quality of research investigating the exercise and mood relationship is acceptable for meaningful conclusions to be generated.

Exercise and Mood: Suggested Mechanisms of Change

Earlier in the chapter, mood was portrayed as transient, fluctuating affective states. The sum of these affective states, namely tension-anxiety, depression-dejection, anger-hostility, vigor-activity, fatigue-inertia, and confusion-bewilderment, produces a composite mood. For this reason, it is very difficult to isolate a specific mechanism (or mechanisms) to explain the exercise and mood relationship. Because of the multidimensional nature of mood, it seems reasonable to assume that any or all of the four exercise and mental health hypotheses outlined in chapter 1 may impact on a participant's mood state. For example, in chapter 2, both the endorphin and monoamine hypotheses were advanced as frequently cited explanations for the exercise and depression relationship. The distraction hypothesis was also depicted as having potential in this regard. Similarly, in chapter 3, both the thermogenic and distraction hypotheses were forwarded as possible explanations for the exercise and anxiety relationship. Because depression-dejection and tension-anxiety are subcomponents of mood state, it is, therefore, reasonable to assume that each of the monoamine, endorphin, thermogenic, and distraction hypotheses has potential to explain the impact of exercise on mood state. Finally, in chapter 4, self-efficacy/skills mastery was discussed as a possible explanation for the exercise and self-concept relationship. Although self-concept/self-esteem is not a specific subcomponent of mood as measured by the POMS, it seems likely that how we feel about ourselves is going to impact on our overall mood (especially positive and negative affect). By mastering physical activity related skills, our self-efficacy is improved, and we consequently feel better about ourselves (i.e., our mood improves). It is important to note that this last position remains conjecture at this point. No research has attempted to examine mood in terms of self-efficacy or skills mastery. It would be interesting for a future study to correlate improvements in self-efficacy with improvements in mood following a specific exercise program. It seems reasonable to expect a significant positive correlation between these two psychological constructs.

Summary and Conclusions

Significant mood improvements have been reported following participation in a wide variety of exercise programs. Most activities appear equally effective in improving mood, although recent evidence suggests greater benefits may result from aerobic exercise. It appears the length of the exercise sessions is not critical in determining the effect of exercise on mood, although longer programs and exercise durations of a minimum of 15 to 20 minutes are recommended. The majority of studies performed suggest exercise must be performed at least three times per week to impact on participant mood. Evidence is now starting to accumulate suggesting that as exercise becomes more intense, mood begins to worsen. Improvements in fitness do not appear necessary for the participant to experience significant positive mood changes. Although all sample populations appear to benefit from an exercise program, individuals with mood problems, such as depression or anxiety, are especially receptive to mood improvements. Because mood is a multidimensional concept, it seems reasonable to assume the monoamine, endorphin, opponent-process, thermogenic, distraction, and self-efficacy/ skills mastery hypotheses all have potential in explaining the exercise and mood relationship.

Suggested Readings

Berger, B.G., & Owen, D.R. (1988). Stress reduction and mood enhancement in four exercise modes: Swimming, body conditioning, hatha yoga, and fencing. *Research Quarterly, 59,* 145-159.

Berger, B.G., Owen, D.R., & Man, F. (1993). A brief review of literature and examination of acute mood benefits of exercise in Czechoslovakian and United States swimmers. *International Journal of Sport Psychology, 24,* 130-150.

Brown, D.R. (1992). Physical activity, ageing, and psychological well-being: An overview of the research. *Canadian Journal of Sports Sciences, 17,* 185-193.

Dyer, J.B., & Crouch, J.G. (1988). Effects of running and other activities on moods. *Perceptual and Motor Skills, 67,* 43-50.

Maroulakis, E., & Zervas, Y. (1993). Effects of aerobic exercise on mood of adult women. *Perceptual and Motor Skills, 76,* 795-801.

McGowan, R.W., Pierce, E., Eastman, N., Tripathi, H.L., Dewey, T., & Olson, K. (1993). Beta-endorphins and mood states during resistance exercise. *Perceptual and Motor Skills, 76,* 376-378.

Moses, J., Steptoe, A., Mathews, A., & Edwards, S. (1989). The effects of exercise training on mental well-being in the normal population: A controlled trial. *Journal of Psychosomatic Research, 33,* 47-61.

Norvell, N., & Belles, D. (1993). Psychological and physical benefits of circuit weight training in law enforcement personnel. *Journal of Consulting and Clinical Psychology, 61,* 520-527.

Chapter 7

EXERCISE ASSESSMENT AND PRESCRIPTION

Readers will immediately recognize that chapter 7 represents a complete change of pace from the earlier chapters. Until this point in time, we have focused our attention almost exclusively upon psychological aspects of the exercise and mental health relationship. In contrast, this chapter examines the exercise component of the association.

The objectives of this chapter are to (a) introduce the basic components of fitness, (b) outline necessary pre-participation screening devices, (c) suggest both laboratory and field assessment techniques for each fitness component, and (d) prescribe appropriate exercise interventions for improving each of these components of fitness.

Specific information of this nature is important for several reasons. First, not everyone who reads this book will be well versed in the exercise assessment and prescription process. In fact, it is likely that only a small percentage represented by exercise physiologists or exercise practitioners will be thoroughly familiar with the concepts presented in the following pages. Some exercise scientists, as well as mental health practitioners and medical personnel, will have had limited exposure to this important information. For this reason, a chapter on exercise assessment and prescription is both appropriate and necessary. Second, exercise is the actual process that impacts either directly or indirectly on mental health. As such, it is important to have a thorough understanding of exercise principles. If exercise is to provide mental health benefits, it must be performed correctly. This chapter will ensure that the exercise prescription process proceeds according to established guidelines. Finally, it is this author's opinion that almost everyone can benefit to some degree by participation in a chronic exercise program. Whereas this book has shown that exercise has significant potential to impact positively on mental health, evidence also exists documenting the positive physiological benefits of chronic participation in physical activity. For this reason, the practitioner who adopts a holistic approach to health would be well advised to prescribe exercise for his or her client. One should keep in mind, however, that the exercise prescription should be performed only by trained professionals.

With this rationale in mind, a brief overview of the different components of fitness will now be provided. This will be followed by specific assessment techniques and prescription principles for each of the individual fitness components.

Basic Components of Fitness

General agreement exists suggesting that fitness involves the four basic components of cardiovascular fitness, muscular strength and endurance, flexibility, and body composition. Depending on the precision required, as well as access to laboratory privileges, a variety of techniques are available that will allow the participant to assess each of these fitness components. The remainder of this chapter will provide an overview of assessment techniques and prescription principles for each of the four components of fitness. In terms of assessment techniques, this chapter will focus on specific field tests that can be performed outside the laboratory setting. For those individuals wishing to utilize more sophisticated measures, several of the more popular laboratory assessments will also be briefly discussed and appropriate references provided.

Pre-Participation Health Screening

Before assessing initial fitness levels and prescribing the actual physical activity program, it is necessary to establish that exercise poses no health risk for a client. Several specific guidelines are provided to assist in this process. The most frequently employed safeguards include the medical examination, the PAR-Q, and contraindications to exercise. Each of these techniques will now be briefly examined.

The medical examination. A medical examination and a diagnostic exercise test should be performed by a physician on males over 40 years of age and females over 50 years of age, even if they are apparently healthy, before starting a vigorous exercise program (American College of Sports Medicine, 1991). However, the American College of Sports Medicine [ACSM] suggests these procedures are not necessary if the participants are beginning a moderate-intensity exercise regimen. For individuals who have been determined to be at higher coronary risk (e.g., hypertensives, people with high cholesterol, smokers, physically inactive people), a maximal exercise test performed by a physician is required. The American College of Sports Medicine (1991) goes on to suggest that for asymptomatic males and females under 40 and 50 years of age respectively for vigorous activity, and apparently healthy individuals of any age for moderate activity, can be effectively screened by means of validated questionnaires. One of the most popular of these questionnaires is the PAR-Q.

   The Physical Activity Readiness Questionnaire. The PAR-Q (British Columbia Department of Health, 1994) was developed in Canada as a pre-exercise screening device. This instrument is illustrated in Figure 7.1. The PAR-Q is believed to be essentially 100% sensitive in detecting medical contraindications to exercise and approximately 80% specific (American College of Sports Medicine, 1991). As such, it has been recommended as a minimum pre-exercise screening device for entry into low-to moderate-intensity exercise programs. Although the PAR-Q is a highly recommended screening tool, it is not without limitations. Shephard (1984), for example, has pointed out that its sensitivity and specificity in predicting subsequent ECG abnormalities are only 30% and 80% respectively. A second criticism of the instrument involves the fact that there is no provision on the form to detect pregnant women or individuals taking prescription medication. Both of these exceptions may alter the safety of exercise. For this reason, the practitioner utilizing the PAR-Q should keep these limitations in mind. For the most part, however, the PAR-Q is an excellent screening device for our purposes. By simply ascertaining that the client is not pregnant or on prescription medication, we can eliminate this limitation. In addition, we have not prescribed vigorous exercise intensity for any of the psychological constructs dealt with in this book. The PAR-Q, therefore, provides an excellent alternative to the medical examination in the majority of cases. But if the client answers yes to any of the seven questions, vigorous exercise and exercise testing should be postponed until clearance is provided by a physician.

   Copies of the PAR-Q can be obtained by writing:

   Government of Canada, Fitness and Amateur Sport

   365 Laurier Avenue West,

   Ottawa, Ontario, CANADA K1A 0X6

   Contraindications for Exercise Training. A final screening method involves checking for contraindications for exercise testing and training. This involves comparing the client's medical history against an established list of contraindications, as illustrated in Table 7.1.

PAR - Q & YOU

Physical Activity Readiness
Questionnaire - PAR-Q
(revised 1994)

(A Questionnaire for People Aged 15 to 69)

Regular physical activity is fun and healthy, and increasingly more people are starting to become more active every day. Being more active is very safe for most people. However, some people should check with their doctor before they start becoming much more physically active.

If you are planning to become much more physically active than you are now, start by answering the seven questions in the box below. If you are between the ages of 15 and 69, the PAR-Q will tell you if you should check with your doctor before you start. If you are over 69 years of age, and you are not used to being very active, check with your doctor.

Common sense is your best guide when you answer these questions. Please read the questions carefully and answer each one honestly: check YES or NO.

YES	NO		
☐	☐	1.	Has your doctor ever said that you have a heart condition <u>and</u> that you should only do physical activity recommended by a doctor?
☐	☐	2.	Do you feel pain in your chest when you do physical activity?
☐	☐	3.	In the past month, have you had chest pain when you were not doing physical activity?
☐	☐	4.	Do you lose your balance because of dizziness or do you ever lose consciousness?
☐	☐	5.	Do you have a bone or joint problem that could be made worse by a change in your physical activity?
☐	☐	6.	Is your doctor currently prescribing drugs (for example, water pills) for your blood pressure or heart condition?
☐	☐	7.	Do you know of <u>any other reason</u> why you should not do physical activity?

If you answered

YES to one or more questions

Talk with your doctor by phone or in person BEFORE you start becoming much more physically active or BEFORE you have a fitness appraisal. Tell your doctor about the PAR-Q and which questions you answered YES.

- You may be able to do any activity you want — as long as you start slowly and build up gradually. Or, you may need to restrict your activities to those which are safe for you. Talk with your doctor about the kinds of activities you wish to participate in and follow his/her advice.
- Find out which community programs are safe and helpful for you.

NO to all questions

If you answered NO honestly to <u>all</u> PAR-Q questions, you can be reasonably sure that you can:

- start becoming much more physically active — begin slowly and build up gradually. This is the safest and easiest way to go.
- take part in a fitness appraisal — this is an excellent way to determine your basic fitness so that you can plan the best way for you to live actively.

DELAY BECOMING MUCH MORE ACTIVE:
- if you are not feeling well because of a temporary illness such as a cold or a fever — wait until you feel better; or
- if you are or may be pregnant — talk to your doctor before you start becoming more active.

<u>Informed Use of the PAR-Q</u>: The Canadian Society for Exercise Physiology, Health Canada, and their agents assume no liability for persons who undertake physical activity, and if in doubt after completing this questionnaire, consult your doctor prior to physical activity.

You are encouraged to copy the PAR-Q but only if you use the entire form

NOTE: If the PAR-Q is being given to a person before he or she participates in a physical activity program or a fitness appraisal, this section may be used for legal or administrative purposes.

I have read, understood and completed this questionnaire. Any questions I had were answered to my full satisfaction.

NAME _____

SIGNATURE _____   DATE _____

SIGNATURE OF PARENT _____   WITNESS _____
or GUARDIAN (for participants under the age of majority)

© Canadian Society for Exercise Physiology
  Société canadienne de physiologie de l'exercice

Supported by: ▮♦▮ Health Santé Canada Canada

continued on other side...

Figure 7.1. The PAR-Q Physical Activity Readiness Questionnaire, used for screening prior to exercise testing and participating in an exercise program. *Note.* From *The PAR-Q Validation Report*, by British Columbia Department of Health, 1978, revised 1994. Copyright © 1994 by Canadian Society for Exercise Physiology. Reprinted by permission.

Table 7.1

Absolute and Relative Contraindications for Exercise Testing and/or Training, used as a Preparticipation Screening Device.

Absolute:
1. Recent myocardial infarction (< 6 weeks)
2. Unstable angina at rest
3. Severe sinus arrhythmias and conduction disturbances
4. Congestive heart failure
5. Aortic stenosis - severe
6. Diagnosed or suspected aortic aneurysm
7. Myocarditis or disease induced cardiomyopathy (recent)
8. Thrombophlebitis, recent emboli (systemic or pulmonary)
9. Fever
10. Uncontrolled metabolic disorders
11. Severe hypertension with exercise (SBP > 250; DBP > 120)

Relative:
1. Frequent ectopic beats and/or uncontrolled supraventricular arrhythmias
2. Pulmonary hypertension - untreated
3. Moderate ventricular aneurysm and/or aortic stenosis
4. Severe myocardial obstructive syndrome
5. Mild cardiomyopathy
6. Toxemia or complicated pregnancy

Conditions requiring a supervised program:
1. Myocardial infarction; postaortocoronary bypass surgery; documented CHD
2. Pacemakers - fixed rate or demand
3. Cardiac medication -chronotropic or inotropic
4. Morbid obesity in conjunction with multiple risk factors
5. ST-Segment depression at rest
6. Severe hypertension
7. Intermittent claudication

Note: From "Exercise Prescription for the Sedentary Adult" by J.M. Goodman and L.S. Goodman, 1985, *Current Therapy in Sports Medicine* (pp. 17-18). Copyright © 1985 by B.C. Decker, Philadelphia. Adapted by permission.

Absolute contraindications for exercise training involve conditions that seriously alter the normal cardiovascular response to exercise. These conditions seriously compromise the client's health. As such, exercise and exercise testing should not be prescribed for individuals thus classified. Relative contraindications require the practitioner to "weigh" the potential benefits of exercise against the associated risks. Clients in this category should be given a supervised exercise test, then enter a supervised program. Medical supervision should be considered mandatory for these clients. Finally, Table 7.1 also lists several contraindications that also require a supervised program. In summary, unless one is a licensed physician, it is advisable to refer the client to a medical doctor if any of the three classifications of contraindications are present in the client.

Now that we have examined three of the most popular pre-participation health screening tools and determined exercise to be safe for our clients, we can devote the remainder of the chapter to exercise assessment and prescription for each of the four basic components of fitness.

Cardiovascular Fitness

Aerobics has become a popular term that illustrates the current fitness craze in North America. A large percentage of people involved in fitness training run, dance, swim, cycle, or skip rope to reap the benefits of improved cardiovascular functioning. A simple definition of cardiovascular fitness is the ability of the heart, lungs, and circulatory system to provide the cells of the body with the substances necessary to sustain work for relatively long periods of time. A variety of tests have been developed to measure cardiovascular fitness. In the next section, we will examine some of the more popular measurement techniques.

Assessing Cardiovascular Fitness

The best and most accurate measure of an individual's cardiovascular fitness is the maximum amount of oxygen the body can use per unit of time (VO2max.). This can be measured very accurately in a laboratory setting or predicted relatively accurately in a field setting.

Laboratory assessment of cardiovascular fitness. An excellent review of laboratory assessment techniques, with normative data and tables depicting the advantages and disadvantages of each testing protocol, is provided by J.

Goodman (1992). Another comprehensive review of these laboratory tests is provided by the American College of Sports Medicine (1991). Both of these reviews suggest treadmill or cycle ergometer testing to determine the most accurate measures of cardiovascular fitness. The reader may consider the above references if he or she has access to state-of-the-art testing equipment. For the most part, however, practitioners will prefer simpler, more cost-efficient tests to determine the client's cardiovascular fitness level. Fortunately, several field tests are available that accomplish this task. In the next section, one particular test that will provide a relatively accurate measure of the client's cardiovascular fitness without complicated and expensive laboratory testing.

Field assessment of cardiovascular fitness. A simple, yet excellent test has been developed by Cooper (1968, 1977) that correlates very well with laboratory measures. The test involves measuring the time spent in running 1.5 miles. The time needed to cover the 1.5 miles is then used to determine the client's fitness level. Despite its simplicity and ease of administration, this field test is almost as accurate and reliable as laboratory measures of gas analysis obtained by treadmill testing (Allsen, Harrison, & Vance, 1989). If a person's fitness level does not allow him or her to participate in the 1.5 mile run, an excellent alternative is provided. A 3- mile walk test will provide the same information without placing as much strain on the client. This is an excellent alternative for individuals who have been physically inactive or are in an older age bracket. The same basic testing steps are followed for either technique. Norms with corresponding fitness levels are provided in Table 7.2.

To perform either of these tests, one should proceed with the following steps:

1. Depending on the client's age and previous level of physical activity, either the 1.5-mile run or the 3- mile walk should be selected.
2. A suitable testing area should be determined. A local high school track is ideal. If a track is not locally available, an appropriate distance on an infrequently used side road may be marked. It is easier to measure out 1/4 mile, than to have the client do round trips over the 1/4 mile distance to cover the necessary mileage.
3. A clock or stopwatch must be available to time the client.
4. The client should warm up by walking, stretching, or performing calisthenics before the testing commences.

Table 7.2

Fitness Norms and Times for the 1.5-Mile Run and the 3.0-Mile Walk

(These tables give times in minutes and seconds.)

1.5-Mile Run Test
Age (years)

Fitness Category		13-19	20-29	30-39	40-49	50-59	60+
I. Very Poor	(men)	>15:31	>16:01	>16:31	>17:31	>19:01	>20:01
	(women)	>18:31	>19:01	>19:31	>20:01	>20:31	>21:01
II. Poor	(men)	12:11-15:30	14:01-16:00	14:44-16:30	15:36-17:30	17:01-19:00	19:01-20:00
	(women)	16:55-18:30	18:31-19:00	19:01-19:30	19:31-20:00	20:01-20:30	20:31-21:00
III. Fair	(men)	10:49-12:10	12:01-14:00	12:31-14:45	13:01-15:35	14:31-17:00	16:16-19:00
	(women)	14:31-16:54	15:55-18:30	16:31-19:00	17:31-19:30	19:01-20:00	19:31-20:30
IV. Good	(men)	9:41-10:48	10:46-12:00	11:01-12:30	11:31-13:00	12:31-14:30	14:00-16:15
	(women)	12:30-14:30	13:31-15:54	14:31-16:30	15:56-17:30	16:31-19:00	17:31-19:30
V. Excellent	(men)	8:37- 9:40	9:45-10:45	10:00-11:00	10:30-11:30	11:00-12:30	11:15-13:59
	(women)	11:50-12:29	12:30-13:30	13:00-14:30	13:45-15:55	14:30-16:30	16:30-17:30
VI. Superior	(men)	< 8:37	<9:45	<10:00	<10:00	<10:30	<11:15
	(women)	< 11:50	<12:30	<13:00	<13:45	<14:30	<16:30

3-Mile Walking Test (No Running)
Age (years)

Fitness Category		13-19	20-29	30-39	40-49	50-59	60+
I. Very Poor	(men)	>45:00	>46:00	>49:00	>52:00	>55:00	>60:00
	(women)	>47:00	>48:00	>51:00	>54:00	>57:00	>63:00
II. Poor	(men)	41:01-45:00	42:01-46:00	44:31-49:00	47:01-52:00	50:01-55:00	54:01-60:00
	(women)	43:01-47:00	44:01-48:00	46:31-51:00	49:01-54:00	52:01-57:00	57:01-63:00
III. Fair	(men)	37:31-41:00	38:31-42:00	40:01-44:30	42:01-47:00	45:01-50:00	48:01-54:00
	(women)	39:31-43:00	40:31-44:00	42:01-46:30	44:01-49:00	47:01-52:00	51:01-57:00
IV. Good	(men)	33:00-37:30	34:00-38:30	35:00-40:00	36:30-42:00	39:00-45:00	41:00-48:00
	(women)	35:00-39:30	36:00-40:30	37:30-42:00	39:00-44:00	42:00-47:00	45:00-51:00
V. Excellent	(men)	<33:00	<34:00	<35:00	<36:30	<39:00	<41:00
	(women)	<35:00	<36:00	<37:30	<39:00	<42:00	<45:00

Note: From The aerobics way, (pp.89-90), by K.H. Cooper, 1977, New York: Copyright by Bantam, Doubleday, Dell. Adapted by permission.

5. The client should be instructed to cover the 1.5 miles (running) or the 3.0 miles (walking) in as fast a time as possible. The client should be instructed to stop immediately if he or she experiences nausea or discomfort.

6. The test time can be used to ascertain the client's fitness category from Table 7.2.

The test is easy to administer and interpret. Periodic evaluation of progress can be determined by comparing this initial fitness level with later scores when the same test is performed at a future date.

Exercise Prescription for Cardiovascular Improvement

Now that the client's initial level of cardiovascular fitness has been determined, it is time to set up an appropriate exercise program to improve this initial score. The following section will describe this important process. This will entail determining the appropriate mode of activity, as well as the exercise intensity, frequency, and duration to ensure maximum benefit for the client.

Mode of exercise. Activities that utilize large muscle groups in a rhythmic and continuous manner are most appropriate for improving cardiovascular fitness (American College of Sports Medicine, 1991; J. Goodman, 1992). In theory, there should be no difference between modes of physical activity in terms of conditioning effect as long as appropriate exercise intensities, frequencies, and durations are met (Fardy, Yanowotz, & Wilson, 1988). These findings suggest that an equal cardiovascular training effect could be gleaned from jogging, swimming, bicycling, cross-country skiing, and aerobic dance. Less intense activities, such as golf and bowling, do not provide the necessary training stimulus to result in cardiovascular fitness gains.

Exercise intensity. It has been suggested that the most difficult problem in designing exercise programs is the prescription of the appropriate exercise intensity (American College of Sports Medicine, 1991). This requires that the exercise program be strictly individualized and monitored to ensure that the maximum prescribed intensity is not exceeded. The most popular methods of prescribing exercise intensity include (a) a percentage of maximum heart rate or heart rate reserve (the maximum minus the resting value) or (b) functional capacity (% of VO2max or metabolic equivalents, or METS). Because of its relative simplicity as well as ease of self-monitoring, the exercise intensity prescription by heart rate is recommended. The practitioner wishing to prescribe intensity by METS is referred to excellent reviews of this technique (American College of Sports Medicine, 1991; J. Goodman, 1992).

Determining exercise intensity by heart rate requires the measurement or estimation of maximal heart rate. Although maximum heart rate can be measured directly in the laboratory following a maximum effort exercise session, this technique is not recommended, due to its potential for health risk. A simpler technique allows us to approximate the client's maximal heart rate by subtracting his or her age from 220. For example, a person 30 years of age would have an estimated maximal heart rate of 190 beats per minute (220 - 30 = 190). A fairly valid and reliable indicator of intensity can be obtained by measuring the heart rate obtained during participation in the physical activity. This can be done by taking the client's pulse. The best location for taking a pulse is over the radial artery on the thumb-side of the wrist. A 10-second pulse is taken immediately (within 5 seconds) following exercise. The first beat is counted as zero, and this observed value is compared to recommended target levels (Figure 7.2). The heart rate necessary to bring about a training effect is between 70% and 85% of the maximal heart rate (American College of Sports Medicine, 1991). To determine the "target heart rate" required for a client to experience a training effect, one should take 70% and 85% of his or her maximal heart rate to find the lowest and highest pulse rates respectively during the exercise session. Using our previous example of a 30-year-old client, this would entail a workout intensity of from 132 to 162 beats per minute. As a simple point of reference for this procedure, Figure 7.2 illustrates the target heart rate zones for clients 20 through 70 years of age (per 10-second and 60-second intervals). This handy chart can be used to prescribe the appropriate exercise intensity for a client.

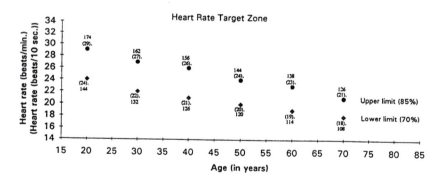

Figure 7.2. The "target zone" for exercise training. Pulse rates (per minute and per 10 seconds) are illustrated, showing the decline in maximal heart rate with age and the corresponding slope of the optimal training intensity with increasing age.

Note. From *CSTF Operations Manual,* 3rd edition, 1987, Health Canada. Copyright © 1994 by the Minister of Supply and Services Canada. Adapted by permission.

Exercise duration. According to the American College of Sports Medicine (1991), a conditioning phase of 20 to 30 minutes of continuous exercise at a moderate intensity is required for the desired training effect to occur. Although a training effect can occur with shorter periods of exercise at higher intensities (J. Goodman, 1992), these high intensity-short duration sessions are not desirable for most participants (American College of Sports Medicine, 1991). In the light of these findings, practitioners are encouraged to prescribe exercise durations of 20 minutes for their clients (30 minutes may be too long for a beginner). This exercise duration closely parallels the duration of exercise recommended to experience improved psychological benefits. This time frame, therefore, appears adequate for both physiological and psychological improvements.

Exercise frequency. The optimal frequency of exercise is dependent upon the intensity and duration of the exercise program. Although a training effect can occur with a frequency of only two sessions per week, the intensity must be relatively high for conditioning to occur (Pollock, 1973). The recommended frequency for normal adults is three sessions per week, with the sessions spaced approximately evenly throughout the week. This is not only the optimal frequency at initial stages of an exercise program, but also allows for sufficient rest between exercise sessions, with sufficient time for musculoskeletal adaptations to occur (American College of Sports Medicine, 1991; J. Goodman, 1992).

Muscular Strength and Endurance

Muscular strength refers to the maximal force (expressed in newtons or kilograms) that can be generated by a particular muscle or muscle group. Muscular endurance, on the other hand, refers to the ability of a specific muscle or muscle group to execute repeated contractions over a period of time that is sufficient to produce muscular fatigue. In our society, many people believe that muscular strength and endurance are important only for athletes or individuals who are required to perform hard manual labour. This is a false assumption. Even the person who works in an office or at home would be better prepared to handle the rigors of day-to-day activities if he or she had an acceptable level of muscular strength and endurance. This becomes even more significant as one reaches 60 years of age or older, when strength has been shown to drop off significantly (Shephard, 1994). In order to determine acceptable levels of these fitness components, several tests have been developed. In the next section, a few of the most popular strength/endurance tests will be reviewed.

Assessing Muscular Strength and Endurance

Techniques used in the assessment of strength and endurance vary considerably. Laboratory tests are available that provide sophisticated data for athletes or for those undergoing neuromuscular and/or musculoskeletal rehabilitation. In addition, simple yet practical field tests have been developed to provide less accurate measures of strength and endurance.

Laboratory assessment of strength and endurance. If one is interested in a sophisticated measure of muscular strength and/or endurance, laboratory tests are available that offer isokinetic assessments. Isokinetic ("constant velocity") strength testing involves the assessment of muscle tension generated throughout an entire range of joint motion at a constant speed (American College of Sports Medicine, 1991). Several commercial companies sell equipment that can provide measures of this nature. This isokinetic equipment can provide an exact measure of concentric muscle contraction, expressed in peak torque (newton-meters or foot pounds). An assessment of muscular endurance can also be provided by selecting an appropriate submaximal level of resistance and counting the number of repetitions performed during a predetermined time limit that would result in muscular fatigue. As mentioned earlier, these laboratory tests are quite sophisticated and are usually reserved for elite athletes or rehabilitation patients. For our purposes, field tests provide a reasonable alternative.

Field assessment of strength and endurance. One popular method of assessing muscular strength is called isotonic strength testing, which refers to muscular contraction against a force (resistance), while allowing muscle shortening. For example, the practitioner may have the client lift the heaviest weight possible in a single attempt (1 RM, or repetition maximum). Free weights or lifting machinery such as the Universal Gym may be used. Jackson, Watkins, and Patton (1980) suggest tests of both upper- and lower-body strength, preferably including the 1 RM bench press (upper body) and 1 RM leg press (lower body). If this strength assessment technique is used, norms are available in a publication entitled *Health/Fitness Instructor's Handbook* (Howley & Franks, 1986). The field tests I recommend for assessing strength and endurance are the ones most commonly utilized, namely the handgrip dynamometer adjusted for hand size and the speed push-ups and sit-ups. The former is a good indicator of muscular strength, whereas the latter provide adequate measures of muscle endurance. A hand dynamometer is a common measurement device that could be borrowed or utilized from most physical education departments at the university and college level. A combined right- and left- hand score (age-specific) is usually reported. Male and female norms for this test are provided in Table 7.3.

Table 7.3
Normative Scores for Push-Ups, Sit-Ups, and Hand Grip Tests of Strength for Males and Females.

Male Norms
Age (Years)

	20-29	30-39	40-49	50-59	60-69
Combined Left and Right Hand Grip (newtons)*					
Excellent	>1129	>1120	>1083	>1000	>927
Above Average	1037-1129	1037-1120	1010-1083	936-1000	854-927
Average	973-1028	963-1028	936-1000	881-927	789-845
Below Average	890-964	890-955	863-927	799-872	725-780
Poor	<890	<890	<863	<799	<725
Push-Ups (total performed)					
Excellent	>35	>29	>21	>20	>17
Above Average	29-35	22-29	17-21	13-20	11-17
Average	22-28	17-21	13-16	10-12	8-10
Below Average	17-21	12-16	10-12	7-9	5-7
Poor	<17	<12	<10	<7	<4
Sit-Ups (total in 60 s)					
Excellent	>42	>35	>31	>26	>23
Above Average	37-42	31-35	26-30	22-25	17-22
Average	33-36	27-30	22-25	18-21	12-16
Below Average	29-32	22-26	17-21	13-17	7-11
Poor	<29	<22	<17	<13	<7

Table 7.3 cont'd...

Female Norms
Age (years)

	20-29	30-39	40-49	50-59	60-69
	Combined Left and Right Grip (newtons)*				
Excellent	>643	>661	>661	>588	>542
Above Average	579-643	606-661	597-661	542-588	496-542
Average	560-588	560-597	542-588	505-532	<568-587
Below Average	505-551	514-551	505-532	468-496	441-459
Poor	<514	<505	<505	<568	<441
	Push-Ups (total performed)				
Excellent	>29	>26	>23	>20	>16
Above Average	21-29	20-26	15-23	11-20	12-16
Average	15-20	13-19	11-14	7-10	5-11
Below Average	10-14	8-12	5-10	2-6	1-4
Poor	<10	<8	<5	<1	<1
	Sit-Ups (total in 60 s)				
Excellent	>35	>28	>24	>18	>15
Above Average	31-35	24-28	20-24	12-18	12-15
Average	25-30	20-23	15-19	5-11	4-11
Below Average	21-24	15-19	7-14	3-4	2-3
Poor	<21	<15	<7	<3	<1

* 1 kg = 9.18 newtons

Note: From CSTF Operations Manual, 3rd edition, Health Canada, 1987.
Reproduced with permission of the Minister of Supply and Services Canada, 1994.

Calisthenic exercise testing has been widely employed to measure muscular endurance. The maximum number of sit-ups performed in one minute and the total number of push-ups performed are counted, then compared to the norms provided in Table 7.3. Males perform the push-ups "straight out," and lower the upper body to a level equal to a fist height above the ground, and must extend with straight arms. For females, the knees are bent and on the floor. The 1-minute speed sit-up test requires the client to perform the maximum number of bent-knee sit-ups possible during the 1-minute duration. During execution, the hands are to be kept locked behind the head. The tester holds the ankles secure while the client sits up touching elbows to knees.

Once again, periodic evaluation of progress can be determined by comparing these initial scores to later measures.

Exercise Prescription for Strength and Endurance

Improvements in muscular strength and endurance are accomplished by means of resistance training, and both involve the principle of overload. There are, however, important differences in prescription. If one wishes to improve muscular strength, the general rule for any exercise is high resistance and a low number of repetitions. To improve muscular endurance, low resistance and a high number of repetitions are desirable. Resistance simply refers to the amount of weight lifted, whereas repetitions involve the number of times the exercise is performed. Let us look at how these principles can be applied to improve a client's strength and endurance.

Mode of exercise. By far the most popular mode of exercise to improve these fitness components is weight lifting, or weight training. Both free weights and lifting machinery, such as the Universal Gym, are widely utilized. To bring about improvements in muscular strength, the client should perform lifts with an amount of weight that he or she can repeat a maximum of six times (6RM, or repetition maximum). The client should follow this same procedure for exercising the different muscle groups. Usually there are 6 to 12 different exercises in a resistance program, utilizing the major muscle groups. A consensus exists that the client should perform 2 or 3 sets (a set is a circuit of all of the exercises in the exercise program). To improve muscular endurance, the client should perform 2 or 3 sets of lifts that can be performed a maximum of 10-12 repetitions. The lower resistance and higher number of repetitions will bring about the desired improvements in muscular endurance. A relatively unique approach to combining strength and endurance is provided by Stone, O'Bryant, and Garhammer (1981). These researchers recommend a step-wise protocol, as follows: (a) 3 weeks of from 3 to 5 sets at 10-20 RM, (b) 4 weeks of 3 sets at 5 RM, and (c) 4 weeks of 3 sets at 3 RM. At the completion of this cycle, either it is repeated, or the individual moves to a maintenance phase. A typical maintenance program would involve 3 sets at 10 RM performed two times per week.

As a general guideline, it is best to exercise large muscle groups before smaller ones. In addition, if the client is exercising for strength improvement, a period of 2-4 minutes between exercises will be required to allow adequate rest and recovery.

Exercise intensity. The concept of exercise intensity for strength and endurance training is closely linked to the preceding section, where resistance and repetitions are prescribed. Two additional tools are available to help you monitor exercise intensity. Earlier in the chapter, practitioners were introduced to the concept of determining the appropriate target heart rate during exercise. As the client becomes familiar with perceiving the appropriate exercise intensity, these pulse rates should be determined once during the exercise session, then immediately after. This will provide a good indication that an appropriate intensity of exercise is being performed. Another valuable technique to monitor exercise intensity is provided by Borg's (1982) Rating of Perceived Exertion (RPE) scale, as illustrated in Table 7.4. These perceived-exertion scales provide a simple method to quantify sub-

Table 7.4

Borg's Rating of Perceived Exertion Scales.

Category RPE Scale		Category-Ratio RPE Scale	
6		0	Nothing at all
7	Very, very light	0.5	Very, very weak
8		1	Very weak
9	Very light	2	Weak
10		3	Moderate
11	Fairly light	4	Somewhat strong
12		5	Strong
13	Somewhat hard	6	
14		7	Very Strong
15	Hard	8	
16		9	
17	Very hard	10	Very, very strong
18		*	Maximal
19	Very, very hard		
20			

Note: From "The Rating of Perceived Exertion" by G.V. Borg, 1982, *Medicine and Science in Sports and Exercise, 14*, p. 377. Copyright © 1982 by Williams & Wilkins. Reprinted by permission.

jective exercise intensity. Scores from the original RPE scale have been shown to correlate closely with several exercise variables, including percent VO2 peak, percent heart rate reserve, minute ventilation, and blood lactate levels (American College of Sports Medicine, 1991; Borg, 1985; J. Goodman, 1992). The linear scale was also developed to provide a more finely tuned subjective response to small increases in objective exercise intensity. The linear scale has been found to be valid for assessing patients with angina. Thus, the original scale is most appropriate for our purposes. As a general guideline, scores of 12-16 on the original scale represent a desirable target heart rate zone for most age groups (Borg, 1985). Use of the RPE scale as an indicator of exercise intensity requires practice. It is unlikely that novice exercisers will have the experience to control their work intensity by purely subjective perceptions. For this reason, in the early stages of an exercise program, one should use the target heart rate method, then gradually introduce the client to the use of the RPE scale.

Frequency and duration. Although 2 days per week can stimulate some changes in muscular strength and endurance, it is generally accepted that 3 days per week is more desirable (American College of Sport Medicine, 1991; J. Goodman, 1992; Howley & Franks, 1986). The actual duration of training can vary considerably, because longer recovery periods are necessary when training for strength development. As a general guideline, however, muscle endurance can be trained for adequately within 20-to 30-minutes sessions, whereas strength development requires approximately 1-hour sessions.

Flexibility

Flexibility is best defined as the maximum ability to move a joint through a complete range of motion. It is concerned with the degree and ease with which the body can twist or bend by means of contracting and relaxing the muscles. There are two main advantages to good flexibility. First, good flexibility results in more efficient movement. In other words, the person spends less energy performing the same task. A second and more important difference is that good flexibility makes the client less vulnerable to injury. Lower-back pain is a condition that is prevalent among both men and women. This problem is considered to be related to a lack of flexibility in the lower back, hips, and hamstrings (upper back of legs), as well as weak abdominal muscles. Another common area of the body that often suffers from lack of flexibility is the upper torso. This section will provide techniques of assessing flexibility, then prescribe appropriate exercises to improve this component of fitness.

Assessing Flexibility

According to J. Goodman (1992), the tests of flexibility fall within two broad categories: direct and indirect measures. For consistency, we will refer to these categories as laboratory and field assessments respectively.

Laboratory assessment of flexibility. The direct measurement of flexibility is most often employed with athletic populations during training or rehabilitation. A goniometer is a protractor-like device and is employed by having the client place the arms along the limbs of the device, then perform a specific physical movement, thus allowing for measurement (in degrees) of flexibility. In addition, an electrogoniometer uses a potentiometer in place of a protractor, thus allowing for flexibility measurement during physical activity. A second direct measure of flexibility may be ascertained by means of a Leighton Flexometer (Leighton, 1955). This instrument involves a device incorporating a rotating needle that is sensitive to gravity. The device is attached to a limb and is capable of measuring the range of motion of a joint in several planes of orientation. This instrument has been shown to have high test-retest reliability and is believed to provide a relatively valid measure of flexibility. Unless one has access to sophisticated equipment of this nature, one will probably employ field tests of flexibility assessment.

Field assessment of flexibility. Admittedly, field tests of flexibility do not provide the degree of accuracy of the more direct laboratory measures. They do, however, provide relatively valid indications of a client's flexibility and, if administered carefully, can be used to monitor progress. There are two field tests of flexibility that are easy to use. These are the Sit-and-Reach Test and the Shoulder-Lift Test (Allsen et al., 1989).

The Sit-and-Reach Test measures the flexibility of the lower back, hips, and the back of the legs (hamstrings). To perform this test, the client should assume a sitting position on the floor. The legs should be placed perpendicular to a line drawn on the floor, with the heels just behind the line. The client's feet should be placed approximately 5 inches apart. A yardstick should be placed on the floor between the client's legs, with the 15-inch mark on the edge of the line nearest the subject's heels. It is best to tape the yardstick to the floor to ensure constant results. Sitting opposite the client, the practitioner can brace heels with his or her own feet. This will prevent the client's feet from slipping over the line. The client should then be instructed to stretch forward and reach, with both hands held together, as far as possible along the yardstick, and hold the position. The score is the farthest point the client can reach on the yardstick with the finger tips. This process is shown in Figure 7.3. The distance should be measured to the nearest inch. This procedure is repeated three times. The best score of the three trials is recorded and compared with the norms provided in Table 7.5.

To perform the Shoulder Lift Test, the client is instructed to lie face down on the floor with the arms extended over the head and a ruler held in both hands. The chin and forehead should maintain contact with the floor during testing. It is also advisable to have someone stabilize the client by placing one hand on the lower back and one on the upper legs. The client is then instructed to raise the arms as high as possible without the rest of the body losing contact with the floor. The distance from the floor that the client is able to raise the ruler is then measured. This is done by having a yardstick resting perpendicular to the floor (or taped to a wall) and measuring the vertical height of the ruler. This process is shown in Figure 7.4. Once again, three trials are given, and the best score recorded. This score can then be compared to the norms illustrated in Table 7.5.

This test is easy to administer and interpret. It is also a valuable resource to test future improvements in the client's flexibility.

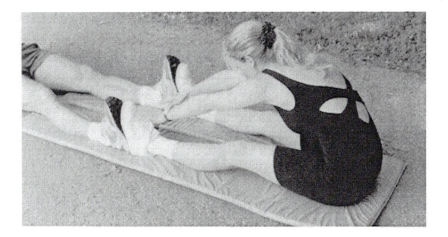

Figure 7.3. The sit-and-reach flexibility test.

Table 7.5

**Flexibility Norms for the Sit-and-Reach test and the
Shoulder Lift Test.**

Sit-and-Reach Flexibility Fitness

Score	Fitness Category
11 or less	Very Poor
12 - 14	Poor
14 - 16	Fair
17 - 19	Good
20 - 21	Very Good
22 - 23	Excellent
24 or more	Superior

Shoulder Lift Flexibility Fitness

Score	Fitness Category
10 or less	Very Poor
11 - 14	Poor
15 - 18	Fair
19 - 21	Good
22 - 24	Very Good
25 - 26	Excellent
27 or more	Superior

Note: From *Fitness for life*, (p. 36), by P.E. Allsen, J.M. Harrison, and B. Vance, 1989, Dubuque, Iowa: Copyright 1989 by W.C. Brown. Adapted by permission.

Exercise Prescription for Flexibility

Increased flexibility is not something that most of us are overly enthusiastic about. Even so, improved flexibility represents a worthwhile goal. We noted earlier that this component of fitness allows us to be more efficient in our movements and to avoid nagging injuries, such as lower-back pain. For this reason, it is important to consider a flexibility component in any exercise program.

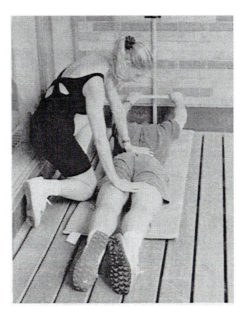

Figure 7.4. The shoulder lift flexibility test.

Mode of exercise. Increased flexibility of the body can be achieved through the proper use of stretching exercises and may involve change in the structure of the ligaments, tendons, and/or musculature. Most stretching exercises are either ballistic (fast, jerky, bobbing movements) or static (slow, sustained movement followed by holding the position). Physiologists have presented a strong case for the superiority of static over ballistic stretching. It is believed that ballistic stretching actually causes the muscle being stretched to tense, thereby causing the muscle to shorten rather than lengthen. Obviously, this effect is counterproductive to what we are trying to accomplish; that is, to stretch or lengthen the muscle under consideration. For this reason, we will focus on static methods of improving flexibility. The following exercises provide a good flexibility training program and involve most of the major muscle groups.

1. The Hamstring Stretch. The client sits with one leg extended on a table, with the opposite leg hanging over the side and resting on the floor. To perform this exercise, the client bends forward at the waist and attempts to touch the toes or beyond. The stretched position should be held for 10 seconds; then the client returns to the starting position. The exercise should

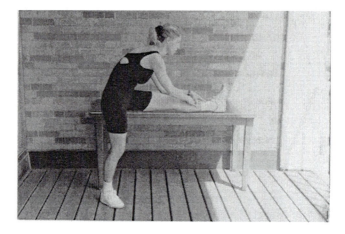

Figure 7.5. The hamstring stretch.

be repeated three times with each leg. This exercise stretches the muscles in the upper-back leg (the hamstrings). See Figure 7.5.

2. The Knee to Chest Curl. The client lies on his or her back and attempts to bring both knees to the chest by grabbing just under the knees and pulling the knees towards the armpits. This position should be held for 10 seconds and repeated three times. This exercise stretches the lower back (low-back extensors). See Figure 7.6.

3. Lying Knee Pull. This exercise is somewhat similar to the previous one, but involves more muscle groups. The client lies on his or her back,

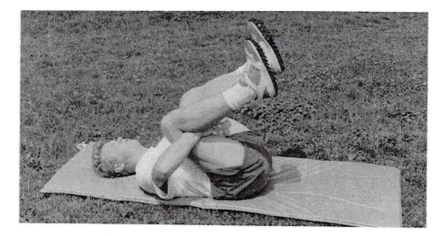

Figure 7.6. The knee to chest curl.

with the legs extended, then brings the left knee to chest, grabbing just under the knee with both hands. It is necessary to pull until a real stretch is felt. This position should be held for 10 seconds; then the client returns to the starting position and performs the same movement with the other leg. These movements should be repeated three times. This exercise stretches the hip flexors, hamstrings, and lower back. See Figure 7.7.

4. Sitting Twist. The client should sit on the floor with legs crossed. The action involves twisting the body to the right, placing the hands on the right side of the thigh and pulling. This movement should be held for 10 seconds; then the client should return to the starting position and repeat the motion to the left. The client should repeat the entire process three times. This exercise is especially valuable for stretching the trunk rotator muscles. See Figure 7.8.

5. Doorframe Stretch. The client stands facing a doorway with hands pointing up and elbows bent at right angles. The hands should rest on the doorframe. The action involves walking slowly through the doorway until stretching is felt in the upper chest. This position should be held for approximately 10 seconds and repeated three times. This exercise stretches the chest muscles (pectoral muscles). See Figure 7.9.

6. Heel-Cord Stretch. The client should initiate this exercise by standing and facing a wall, with the palms against the wall and the body at arm's length. The feet should be spread slightly apart. Keeping the feet flat, the client leans forward allowing the elbows to bend slightly until stretching is felt in the calf muscles. This position should be held for 10 seconds and

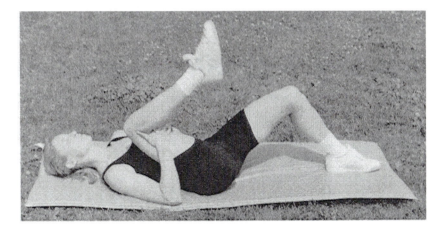

Figure 7.7. The lying knee pull.

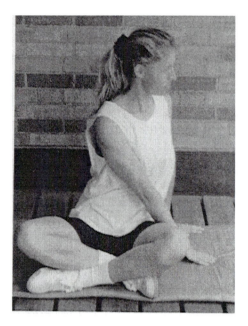

Figure 7.8. The sitting twist.

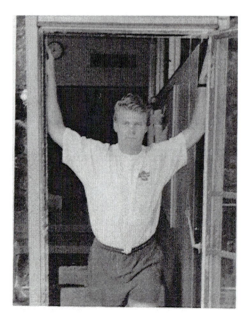

Figure 7.9. The doorframe stretch.

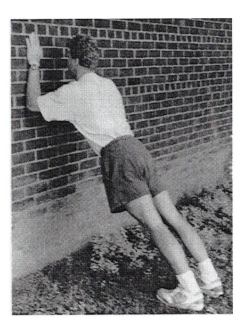

Figure 7.10. The heel-cord stretch.

repeated three times. This exercise is valuable for stretching the heel cord and calf muscles (achilles tendon, gastrocnemius, and soleus (see Figure 7.10).

Exercise frequency. To be effective, a flexibility program should be performed daily. If this is not possible, the practitioner should at least try to have the client stretch three or four times per week. Stretching may be done as an exercise program in itself or included after an aerobic or anaerobic workout.

Guidelines for stretching. A comprehensive set of guidelines for stretching is provided by Allsen et al. (1989, pp. 156-157). These include (a) stretch daily, because it takes considerable time to improve flexibility, (b) warm up the muscles gradually before doing any of the stretching exercises, (c) perform the stretching exercise slowly and continue until stretch on the muscle is felt, (d) avoid pain, because it is not part of a good stretching program, (e) hold the stretch position for at least 10 seconds, (f) relax the muscle that is being placed in a stretched position, (g) release slowly from this stretched position. We should remember that developing a safe and effective stretching program necessitates careful planning. It will, however, pay valuable dividends as part of a total fitness program.

Body Composition

The evaluation of body composition is usually included as part of any overall fitness assessment. During the past several decades there has been a change in the cultural norm of what people think the ideal body should look like. Unfortunately, the slender bodies of models and movie superstars have become the ideal that many individuals strive for, either consciously or unconsciously. Most people realize that excessive body fat is harmful to the health. Not nearly as many realize that not enough weight can also pose health risks. To determine appropriate weight for any individual, a variety of assessment techniques exist. Once again, both laboratory and field assessments are available.

Laboratory assessment of body composition. Body composition refers to the percentage of body weight that is fat (% body fat). It is based on the assumption that both lean body weight and fat body weight are included in our body composition. The most popular laboratory measure of body composition is hydrostatic (underwater) weighing (Brozek & Keys, 1951). This technique is based on Archimedes' principle that when a body is immersed in water, it will be buoyed up by a counterforce equal to the weight of water displaced. Because bone and muscle are denser than fat, a person with more lean body mass will weigh more in water, and hence have a lower percentage of body fat. Although this technique is the ultimate assessment for body composition, it requires special and sophisticated equipment and is, therefore, of little use to the practitioner. Fortunately, relatively simple field tests are also available that give us a good estimate of body composition.

Field assessment of body composition. The most popular field tests to assess body compositon include anthropometric measures, skinfold thickness, and circumference measurements. These assessment techniques are fully explained in recent reviews (American College of Sports Medicine, 1991; J. Goodman, 1992; Howley & Franks, 1986). The field test recommended for your purposes is referred to as the Body Mass Index (Health and Welfare Canada, 1988). This index is calculated by dividing body weight in kilograms by weight in meters squared. Fortunately, this figure can be ascertained easily without the frightening mathematics. We can simply refer to Figure 7.11 to calculate a client's BMI score. To determine BMI from Figure 7.11, we mark an X at the client's height on line A, then mark an X at the client's weight on line B. Then we take a ruler and join the two Xs. To find the client's BMI, we extend this line to line C. For example, a person

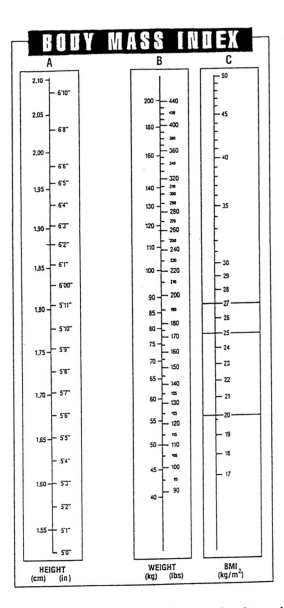

Figure 7.11. The Body Mass Index (BMI) Scale, used to determine a healthy body.

Note. From "The Body Mass Index" by Health Canada, 1991. Copyright © 1994 by the Minister of Supply and Services Canada. Reprinted by permission

who is 5'10" tall and weighs 175 pounds would have a BMI of between 25 and 26. Once we have calculated the client's BMI, we can compare it to the following established norms (Health and Welfare Canada, 1988):

Under 20: A score under 20 may be associated with health problems for some individuals. The client should consult a physician or dietician.

20 - 25: This zone is associated with the lowest risk of illness for most people. This is the range the client should stay in.

25 - 27: This range may be associated with health problems for some individuals. The client should be encouraged to lose some weight.

Over 27: A BMI over 27 is associated with increased health risk. The client should consult his or her physician for advice.

In summary, the BMI is an excellent indicator of total body composition and has been found to relate very well to health outcomes. It is easy to use and can provide a target weight range for a client if he or she is not already in the 20-25 BMI range.

Exercise Prescription for Body Composition

Body composition is determined by a complex set of genetic and behavioral factors. Although the contributing factors are many, the key to managing weight effectively is simply the balance of calories consumed versus those expended. In other words, caloric intake refers to the energy equivalent of food ingested, whereas caloric expenditure involves the energy equivalent of work performed. It is an established fact that one pound of fat is the equivalent of approximately 3,500 kilocalories (kcal) of energy. This means that if caloric intake remains the same, a client must burn 3,500 kcal of energy to lose one pound of body fat. We can soon see that losing weight by exercise alone is a very slow process indeed. The best way to lose weight is to take in fewer kilocalories per day in one's diet, while expending more energy by means of an appropriate exercise program. As a general recommended guideline, the maximum rate of weight loss should never exceed 1.0 to 1.5 pounds per week. Although specific dietary advice is beyond the scope of this book, a few specific guidelines will help the practitioner to balance the diet and exercise equation with the client. To determine the client's average caloric intake per day, it is necessary to have a record of everything he or she eats and drinks during an average week. It may even be a good idea to continue this recording for a baseline of two weeks. Most bookstores and supermarkets have easy-to-use booklets that illustrate the kilocalories of common foods. The Allsen et al. (1989) reference mentioned earlier is an excellent example of a such a book. By determining a client's average kcal intake, it will be possible to determine a suitable reduction that can be used as one step in the weight loss program (i.e., the ubiquitous diet). The second step, and the one we are primarily interested in with this publication, is the process of increasing caloric expenditure on a day-to-day basis. In the following section, we will look at common kcal expenditures of different modes of exercise. We should remember that losing weight involves a combination of eating less and exercising more. For example, simple mathematics tells us that if we eat 250 kcal less per day and expend 250 more kcal per day through exercise, this will result in a net balance of -500 kcal/day. At the end of one week, this would produce an actual weight loss of one full pound (500kcal x 7 = 3,500 kcal). There is nothing magical about this formula. The only thing we must remember is that we take in fewer kilocalories each week than usual and expend more kilocalories than usual. This simple approach will help a client lose unwanted weight. It should be noted that we have not considered the client's basal metabolic rate or the amount of energy needed to maintain the body at rest. If we follow the earlier simple guideline, we need not concern ourselves with this concept. The goal is to for the client to develop a negative energy balance by eating less and exercising more than he or she has in the past. Now that we have briefly discussed the role of diet, let us look at the role of exercise in weight loss.

Mode of exercise. Obviously, different exercise modes will have different kilocaloric expenditures. The more vigorous the activity, the greater the potential weight loss. An excellent summary of energy requirements for several physical activities is provided in Table 7.6. To illustrate the practical significance of the information presented in this section, let us consider the following example. A client named Bob has completed the BMI index and figures he needs to lose 5 pounds from his current weight of 163 pounds. Because the client knows that one pound of body fat is the equivalent of 3,500 kcal, he realizes this goal corresponds to a net loss of 17,500 kcal (5 x 3500 = 17,500 kcal). To reach this goal, the practitioner recommends the following:

1. Every day of the week, the client will walk for 30 minutes. This will lead to a total daily expenditure of 177 kcal (5.9 kcal/min x 30 minutes). Because Bob has been physically inactive in the past, this will be a net loss of 177 kcal per day.

Table 7.6

Energy Requirements (kcal/min) for Several Physical Activities, Used to Allow the Participant to Calculate Energy Expenditures for a Given Workout.

Activity (kcal/min/kg)*	130 lb.	163 lb.
Calisthenics (0.73)	4.3	5.4
Cycling		
5.5 mph (.064)	3.8	4.7
Golf (0.85)	5.0	6.3
Racquetball (.143)	8.4	10.6
Running		
Cross-country (.163)	9.1	12.1
9 min/mi (.193)	11.4	14.3
7 min/mi (.228)	13.9	16.8
Swimming		
Slow crawl (.128)	7.6	9.5
Fast crawl (.156)	9.2	11.5
Tennis (.109)	6.4	8.1
Walking		
Normal (.080)	4.7	5.9
Weight Training (.116)	6.8	8.6

* To calculate the kcal expenditure for subjects whose weight is not close to 130 or 163 lb., simply convert their body weight to kilograms and multiply this figure by the values given in parentheses.

Note: From *Fitness motivation: Preventing participant drop-out* (p. 65), by W.J. Rejeski, and E.A. Kenney, 1988, Champaign, Illinois: Copyright © 1988 by Life Enhancement Publications, a division of Human Kinetics. Reproduced by permission.

2. In terms of diet, Bob feels he can do without his before dinner cocktail each evening, resulting in a net daily loss of 200 kcal (the calories in an average cocktail).

3. The previous two points result in a net negative balance of 377 kcal per day (177 kcal from exercise + 200 kcal from diet).

4. By dividing 17,500 kcal by 377 (the number of calories expended through exercise and diet), Bob calculates that it will take approximately 46

days to lose 5 pounds. This means that in a little over 6 weeks, Bob will reach his goal.

Summary and Conclusions

This chapter has presented the four basic components of fitness. I have recommended specific field tests to measure each component and outlined exercise prescription principles for improving the specific component of fitness under consideration. Throughout the book, a variety of exercise prescription guidelines for improving the psychological construct under consideration have been provided. In all cases, I have followed the assessment and prescription principles outlined in this chapter. One should keep in mind, however, that it was necessary to prescribe exercise modes based upon information gleaned from completed research. In all cases, an attempt was made to match the appropriate exercise mode with the appropriate psychological construct. In other words, the primary objective was enhancing mental health by means of exercise. Exercise in this manner can be seen as a means towards an end, and not an end in itself. Nevertheless, it was still important to follow established exercise principles. Hence, chapter 7 has been included as a set of guidelines for prescribing appropriate exercise for your clients. It represents the latest information available to assist practitioners in their important endeavors.

Suggested Readings

Allsen, P.E., Harrison, J.M., & Vance, B. (1989). *Fitness for life*. Dubuque, IA: Wm. C. Brown.

American College of Sports Medicine. (1983). Position statement on proper and improper weight loss program. *Medicine and Science in Sports and Exercise, 15*, ix-xiii.

American College of Sports Medicine. (1991). *Guidelines for exercise testing and prescription*. Philadelphia: Lea & Febiger.

Goodman, J. (1992). Assessment of exercise capacity and principles of exercise prescription. In R.J. Shephard & H.S. Miller (Eds.), *Exercise and the heart in health and disease* (pp. 55-103). New York: Marcel Dekker, Inc.

Howley, E.T., & Franks, B.D. (1986). *Health/fitness instructor's handbook*. Champaign, IL: Human Kinetics.

Shephard, R.J. (1994). *Aerobic fitness & health.* Champaign, IL.: Human Kinetics.

Stone, M.H., O'Bryant, H., & Garhammer, J. (1981). A hypothetical model for strength training. *Journal of Sports Medicine and Physical Fitness, 21,* 342-351.

Chapter 8

PRESENT STATUS AND FUTURE DIRECTIONS

Now that we have reviewed the empirical literature investigating the effects of exercise on several aspects of mental health, **the objectives of this chapter are to (a) summarize the current state of knowledge, (b) suggest some problematic issues in studying the exercise and mental health relationship, and (c) provide some direction for future research.**

Conclusions: Current Status

On the basis of completed research, it appears the following conclusions regarding the exercise and mental health relationship are warranted:

1. Exercise is consistently associated with improvements in the psychological states of depression, state anxiety, and mood.

2. Psychological traits, such as global personality, self-concept/self-esteem, and trait anxiety, have been subject to modest improvements following involvement in a prolonged exercise program. These results are less consistent than those involving psychological states.

3. In regard to type of exercise, aerobic, anaerobic and nonaerobic activities appear equally effective in producing positive mental benefits, although isolated studies suggest aerobic exercise is most effective. Within these respective categories, no single type of exercise has been shown to be superior, although running has been the most frequently studied activity.

4. The optimal exercise frequency, intensity, and duration required to produce the greatest psychological benefits have not been clearly established. Trends are provided for each psychological construct as **prescription guidelines** in the respective chapters.

5. Improved physical fitness does not appear to be a prerequisite for improved psychological benefits.

6. Exercise appears to have beneficial psychological effects across all ages, sexes, and sample populations.

7. Exercise appears as effective in treating mental disorders as the more traditional therapies, such as psychotherapy, meditation, cognitive therapy, and relaxation, although it should not be used independently without medical, psychological, or psychiatric clearance.

8. The exact mechanism explaining the exercise and mental health relationship has not been clearly established, although the endorphin, monamine, thermogenic, and distraction hypotheses have received the greatest attention in the literature.

Exercise and Mental Health: Possible Detrimental Effects

The research reviewed up to this point in the monograph has dealt almost exclusively with positive effects of exercise on mental health. However, recent research is focusing increased attention on the possibility that exercise may also be associated with negative psychological changes in the participant (Biddle & Fox, 1989; D.R. Brown, 1990; Kirkcaldy & Shephard, 1990; Morgan & Goldston, 1987; Morgan & O'Connor, 1989; Raglin, 1990, 1993; Veale, 1991).

Exercise Abuse

An article by Morgan and O'Connor (1989) outlines a syndrome referred to as exercise abuse. These researchers suggest that individuals who are exercise abusers typically place an inordinately high priority on physical activity. A person characterized by this syndrome often displays an unwillingness to quit exercising even in the face of medical injury. Similarly, a small proportion of these individuals will train to such an extent that exercise results in negative social and career consequences (D.R. Brown, 1990; Morgan, 1979b, 1979c; Raglin, 1990). In addition, a small number of highly dedicated runners have also been found to suffer from eating disorders (Katz, 1986). At present, information on exercise abuse is primarily descriptive. Research is now required to establish its etiology and prevalence (Raglin, 1990).

Exercise Addiction

An interesting corollary to the exercise abuse syndrome involves the concept of exercise addiction. Exercise addiction may be either positive or negative. The concept of a positive addiction to exercise, and running in particular, was popularized by Glasser (1976) in his book *Positive Addiction*. At the same time, Kostrabula (1976) also suggested the positively addicting aspects in his book *The Joy of Running*. Glasser's (1976) book is essentially an analysis of addictions which he views as supportive of the addict's physiology and psychology. Glasser views activities, such as meditation and running, to be positive addictions. Positive addictions were thought to provide psychological strength and increase an individual's satisfaction with life. Negative addictions such as alcohol or heroin, on the other hand, weaken or undermine both physiological and psychological integrity. The work of Glasser is not scientifically based in the sense of rigorous experimental design. The use of clinical and psychiatric assessments, however, provides useful anecdotes. Exercisers typically report feeling "high" or "euphoric" after a workout. Classic descriptions of this positive addiction state include such terms as (a) floating, (b) euphoria, (c) loss of the sense of oneself, and (d) total integration with exercise. This runner's high has been further defined by Sachs (1980) as a euphoric, usually unexpected, sensation experienced during running, usually unexpected, in which the runner feels a heightened sense of well-being, enhanced appreciation of nature, and transcendence of barriers of time and space.

Although it has been suggested that some regular exercisers, such as joggers, may actually become addicted to the running experience (Morgan, 1979b; Peele, 1981; Yates, Leehey, & Slisslak, 1983), the results of this addiction may not always be positive. An excellent study by Yates et al. (1983) highlights this point. On the basis of interviews with marathoners and trail runners, the researchers concluded that the running experience preempts all other interests in life. These same researchers reported that exercise deprivation was observed to produce depression and anxiety in obligatory runners. In addition, other studies have shown that the inability to pursue the high level of physical activity to which an individual has become accustomed can lead to negative psychological states, including feelings of hostility, headache, frustration, and tension (Glasser, 1976), as well as restlessness, irritability, and guilt (Robbins & Joseph, 1985). Incidences of this nature point out the potential of exercise's becoming a negative addiction. In other studies, this phenomenon has been labeled runner's gluttony, fitness fanaticism, athlete's neurosis, and obligatory running (Dishman, 1985).

The positive/negative addiction distinction is an important one. In positive addiction, the individual controls the exercise environment. On the other hand, as Morgan (1979b, 1979c) points out, for some individuals, exercise controls them. For these people, exercise has become a negative addiction. As Sachs (1984a) has pointed out, it is probably best not to use the term *addiction* when discussing the positive relationship between an individual and exercise. Addiction implies controlling an individual to the extent that it hurts his or her functioning. Although this is the case with negative addiction, it is certainly not the case in positive addiction. The running guru Sheehan (1983) agrees, arguing that the term addiction should not be used to explain exercise behavior. He feels the terms *commitment* or *dedication* are more appropriate. Peele (1981) supports this position, suggesting that no evidence has been provided indicating that exercise addicts differ neurologically from nonaddicted exercisers. As a compromise, Peele has suggested the term *healthy habits* to characterize activities such as exercise, especially when exercise enhances the person's feeling of control over personal well-being. Regardless of whether we use the term addiction or healthy habits, exercise is still praised as a behavior with potential to improve an individual's quality of life. For a more thorough review of the addiction controversy, the reader is referred to Morgan (1979b, 1988) and Sachs (1981, 1984a).

Overtraining and Staleness

Another possible negative outcome of exercise has been referred to as the staleness syndrome (Morgan et al., 1987; Ryan, 1983; Veale, 1991). In an attempt to enhance performance, endurance athletes (e.g., distance runners, swimmers) often engage in periods of intensified training, or overtraining. Overtraining usually lasts for several weeks, then is followed by large reductions in training, or tapering. Morgan et al. (1987) have shown that overtraining is associated with increases in mood disturbance, with mood disturbance becoming progressively worse as training intensifies, then becoming progressively better as training tapers. A 10-year longitudinal study by Morgan et al., (1988) monitored over 200 male and 200 female swimmers involved in competitive swimming. In a series of studies, they found that (a) there is a dose-response relationship, with significant increases in training associated with significant increases in mood disturbance; (b) early psychological indicators of overtraining as measured by the POMS include increases in fatigue and decreases in vigor, with negative changes in depression, tension, and anger as chronic overtraining continues; and (c) the monitoring of individual mood profiles may serve as an early warning system for the onset of staleness. The latter point is especially important from a practical perspective. A future study employing an A-B-A single subject repeated-measures design should be performed to determine the effect of psychological monitoring and tapering on performance. The early work by Morgan et al. (1987, 1988) suggests psychological monitoring is capable of detecting early symptoms of staleness, which could then be followed by immediate tapering. An experiment of this nature should therefore demonstrate significant improvements in performance, rather than the previously reported drop-offs due to staleness.

The only known cure for staleness is rest. Many stale athletes may need to cease training for several weeks. Although staleness is mainly confined to competitive/elite athletes, at least one study suggests it can occur in recreational athletes as well (Yates et al., 1983).

Investigation of the detrimental as well as the beneficial psychological consequences of exercise is necessary if we are to thoroughly understand the exercise and mental health relationship. Information of this nature not only expands our knowledge, but also has practical value in maximizing the psychological benefits of exercise for elite athletes in addition to the more often studied normal and clinical samples.

Future Directions

Although the field of exercise and mental health is expanding rapidly, a great deal remains to be learned about the nature of the relationship. Although specific recommendations have been provided throughout this manuscript, this final section outlines several directions for research that have potential to further our understanding.

1. A great deal of attention in recent literature reviews has focused on methodological problems inherent in the completed research (D.R. Brown, 1990; Doan & Scherman, 1987; Kirkcaldy & Shephard, 1990; Leith & Taylor, 1990; Sime, 1990). For example, a large proportion of the exercise and mental health literature consists of descriptive, correlational, and cross-sectional studies. Very few true experimental studies possessing good internal and external validity have been performed. For this reason, it is not possible to unequivocally infer a causal relationship between exercise and mental health. Other common methodological problems that must be remedied include (a) nonrandom assignment of subjects to groups and groups to treat-

ments, (b) failure to control for a Hawthorne effect by means of placebo and/ or true control group treatment conditions, and (c) failure to utilize double-blind research designs. An excellent resource for controlling methodological problems of this nature is provided by Campbell and Stanley (1963) in their classic research design text *Experimental and Quasi-experimental Designs for Research.* Researchers would be well advised to consult this publication in determining an appropriate research design. Finally, there is need for more longitudinal research, because the psychological effects of exercise may accumulate or diminish over time.

2. A second problematic area involves getting those people involved in exercise who need it most. Extensive surveys (Fitness Canada, 1986; Harris, 1979; Sports Council, 1982) have shown that at best, only approximately one-half the population take part in regular exercise, and of those who do, only a small number exercise in a manner that results in fitness gains or health benefits of any magnitude. Along similar lines, personal experience tells us that when we are depressed or upset about something, this is the time we feel least like exercising. This problem is of an even greater magnitude when we are dealing with clinically symptomatic (e.g., anxious, depressed) individuals. A new branch of research should be developed involving exercise as a motivational issue. Collaborative research efforts with the field of psychology could investigate current motivational theory and apply it to participation in chronic exercise programs. By identifying the proper motivational techniques, individuals could be more adequately enticed to exercise. Concomitantly, they will experience the ensuing physiological and psychological benefits.

3. An effort should be made to combine exercise and mental health research with exercise adherence research. Once we have attracted participants to an exercise program, how can we best ensure long-term involvement? This consideration is an important one. Research has demonstrated approximately 50% of those individuals engaging in an exercise program will drop out within the first 3 to 6 months (Dishman, 1982; J.E. Martin & Dubbert, 1982; Oldridge, 1982). Because exercise has been demonstrated to impact positively on mental health, the maintenance of an exercise program would increase the chances of lasting psychological benefits. A recent review by Leith and Taylor (1992) highlights a variety of behavioral techniques shown to be associated with significant improvements in exercise adherence. Behavior change strategies, such as contracting, behavioral contingencies, self-recording, cost-benefit analysis, stimulus cueing, goal set-

ting, and social reinforcement, have all been found to improve exercise adherence (Leith & Taylor, 1992). By including these exercise adherence principles in the research design, the probability will be enhanced that the participants will remain in the exercise program. Future studies should also employ follow-up measures (e.g., 3-month, 6-month, 1-year) to determine if the exercise program has been maintained, and hence the psychological benefits still manifest.

4. Because of contemporary funding and program limitations, research should attempt to focus on individual life-style activities that could be performed without the need for a formal setting. An aerobic activity, such as walking, for example, can be performed at a minimum expense in most locations. Future research should, therefore, attempt to provide some guidelines regarding the "how often" and "how long" of this type of activity. This is not to ignore the possible benefits of other forms of exercise. Many additional physical activities, especially those involving a social component, have significant potential to impact on mental health. The suggestion here is to devote more research attention to a type of exercise that is most practical, affordable, and expedient to the participant.

5. In conclusion, one final point warrants consideration. The opportunity now exists for exercise scientists and mental health practitioners to focus on an exercise and wellness relationship. The majority of research conducted to date has primarily involved treating or improving a psychological disorder or construct. A whole new line of research should now examine the potential of exercise in the prevention of such disorders. Longitudinal studies, performed over several years, could compare samples of regular exercisers and nonexercisers in terms of the incidence of mental disorders. On the basis of research utilizing nonclinical populations examined in *Foundations of Exercise and Mental Health*, it seems reasonable to assume that exercise will serve a viable function in the promotion of mental health in the participant.

Finally, much more research is needed to determine the mechanisms responsible for exercise-induced changes in mental health. Future collaboration with exercise biochemists is needed to enhance our understanding of the biochemical mechanisms underlying the exercise and mental health relationship.

Suggested Readings

Biddle, S.J., & Fox, K.R. (1989). Exercise and health psychology: Emerging relationships. *British Journal of Medical Psychology, 62,* 205-216.

Kirkcaldy, B.D., & Shephard, R.J. (1990). Therapeutic implications of exercise. *International Journal of Sport Psychology, 21,* 165-184.

Morgan, W.P., & O'Connor, P.J. (1989). Psychological effects of exercise and sports. In E. Ryan & R. Allman (Eds.), *Sports medicine* (pp. 671-689). New York: Academic Press.

Raglin, J.S. (1990). Exercise and mental health: Beneficial and detrimental effects. *Sports Medicine, 9,* 323-329.

Raglin, J.S. (1993). Overtraining and staleness: Psychometric monitoring of endurance athletes. In R.N. Singer, M. Murphy, & L.K. Tennant (Eds.), *Handbook of research on sport psychology* (pp. 840-850). New York: Macmillan.

Veale, D.M.W. (1991). Psychological aspects of staleness and dependence on exercise. *International Journal of Sports Medicine, 12,* 19-22.

References

Abadie, B.R. (1987). The physiological and psychological effects of an endurance exercise program on an older adult population (Doctoral dissertation, University of Southern Mississippi, 1986). *Dissertation Abstracts International, 47*, 3693-A.

Adler, A. (1929). *The practice and theory of individual psychology.* New York: Brace & World.

Akiskal, H.S., & McKinney, W.T. (1975). Overview of recent research in depression: Integration of ten conceptual models into a comprehensive clinical frame. *Archives of General Psychiatry, 32*, 285-305.

Allport, G.W. (1937). *Basic considerations for psychology of personality.* New Haven: Yale University Press.

Allsen, P.E., Harrison, J.M., & Vance, B. (1989). *Fitness for life.* Dubuque, IA: Wm. C. Brown.

American College of Sports Medicine. (1983). Position statement on proper and improper weight loss program. *Medicine and Science in Sports and Exercise, 15*, ix-xiii.

American College of Sports Medicine. (1991). *Guidelines for exercise testing and prescription.* Philadelphia: Lea & Febiger.

American Psychiatric Association (1980). *Diagnostic and statistical manual of mental disorders* (2nd ed.). Washington, D.C.

American Psychiatric Association (1987). *Diagnostic and statistical manual of mental disorders* (3rd ed.). Washington, D.C.

Andres, F.F., Metz, K.F., & Drash, A.L. (1978). Changes in state anxiety and urine catecholamines produced during treadmill running. *Medicine and Science in Sports and Exercise, 10*, 51.

Angyal. A.A. (1951). Theoretical model for personality studies. *Journal of Personality, 20*, 137-149.

Appenzeller, O. (1980, July). Report from Otto Appenzeller, M.D., *T h e AMJA Newsletter*, p. 31.

Appenzeller, O. (1981a, August). Does running affect mood? (In Reader's Forum), *Runner's World, 16*, p. 13.

Appenzeller, O. (1981b). What makes us run? *New England Journal of Medicine, 305*, 578-580.

Appenzeller, O., & Schade, D.R. (1979). Neurology of endurance training III: Sympathetic activity during a marathon run. *Neurology, 29,* 542.

Appenzeller, O., Standefer, J., Appenzeller, J., & Atkinson, R. (1980). Neurology of endurance training V: Endorphins. *Neurology, 30,* 418-419.

Atkins, C.J., Kaplan, R.M., Timms, R.M., Reinsch, S., & Lofback, K. (1984). Behavioral exercise programs in the management of chronic obstructive pulmonary disease. *Journal of Consulting and Clinical Psychology, 52,* 591-603.

Auweele, Y.V., DeCuyper, B., Van Mele, V., & Rzewnicki, R. (1993). Elite performance and personality: From description and prediction to diagnosis and intervention. In R. Singer, M. Murphy, & L. Tennant (Eds.), *Handbook of research on sport psychology* (pp. 257-289). New York: Macmillan.

Bahrke, M.S., & Morgan, W.P. (1978). Anxiety reduction following exercise and meditation. *Cognitive Therapy and Research, 2,* 323-333.

Balog, L. (1983). The effects of exercise muscle tension and subsequent muscle relaxation training. , 119-125.

Bandura, A. (1962). Social learning through imitation. In M.R. Jones (Ed.), *Nebraska symposium on motivation* (pp. 76-108. Lincoln, NE: University of Nebraska Press.

Bandura, A. (1965). Influence of model's reinforcement contingencies on the acquisition of imitative responses. *Journal of Personality and Social Psychology, 1,* 589-595.

Bandura, A. (1969). *Principles of behavior modification.* New York: Holt, Rinehart & Winston.

Bandura, A. (1977). Self-efficacy: Toward a unifying theory of behavioral change. *Psychological Review, 84,* 191-215.

Bandura, A. (1982). Self-efficacy mechanism in human aging. *American Psychologist, 37,* 122-147.

Barchas, J., & Freedman, D. (1962). Brain amines: Response to physiological stress. *Biochemical Pharmacology, 12,* 1232-1235.

Bar-Eli, M., & Tenenbaum, G. (1988). The interaction of individual psychological crisis and time phases in basketball. *Perceptual and Motor Skills, 66,* 523-530.

Bar-Eli, M., & Tenenbaum, G. (1989). Game standings and psychological crisis in sport: Theory and research. *Canadian Journal of Sport Sciences, 4,* 31-37.

Barlow, D.H. (1988). *Anxiety and its disorders: The nature and treatment of anxiety and panic.* New York:Guilford Press.

Baron, R.A., Byrne, D., & Kantowitz, B. (1980). *Psychology: Understanding behavior* (2nd ed.). New York: Holt, Rinehart & Winston.

Barrett, C. (1980). Personality character disorders. In R. Woody (Ed.), *The encyclopedia of clinical assessment.* San Francisco: Jossey-Bass.

Beck, A.T., Ward, C.H., Mendelson, M., Mock, J. & Erbaugh, J. (1961). An inventory for measuring depression. *Archives of General Psychiatry, 4,* 561-571.

Beckman, H., Ebert, M.H., Post, R., & Goodwin, E.K. (1979).Effects of moderate exercise on urinary MHPG in depressed patients. *Pharmakopsychiatry, 12,* 351-356.

Ben-Schlomo, L.S., & Short, M.A. (1986). The effects of physical conditioning on selected dimensions of self-concept in sedentary females. *Occupational Therapy in Mental Health, 5,* 27-46.

Berger, B.G. (1984). *Running as therapy: An integrated approach.* Lincoln, NE: University of Nebraska Press.

Berger, B.G. (1994). Coping with stress: The effectiveness of exercise and other techniques. *Quest, 46,* 100-119.

Berger, B.G., Friedman, E., & Eaton, M. (1988). Comparison of jogging, the relaxation response, and group interaction for stress reduction. *Journal of Sport and Exercise Psychology, 10,* 431-437.

Berger, B.G., & Owen, D.R. (1983). Mood alteration with swimming: Swimmers really do "feel better." *Psychosomatic Medicine, 45,* 425-431.

Berger, B.G., & Owen, D.R. (1987). Anxiety reduction with swimming: Relationships between exercise and state, trait, and somatic anxiety. *International Journal of Sport Psychology, 18,* 286-302.

Berger, B.G., & Owen, D.R. (1988). Stress reduction and mood enhancement in four exercise modes: Swimming, body conditioning, hatha yoga, and fencing. *Research Quarterly, 59,* 145-159.

Berger, B.G., & Owen, D.R. (1992). Preliminary analysis of a causal relationship between swimming and stress reduction: Intense exercise may negate the effects. *International Journal of Sport Psychology, 23,* 70-85.

Berger, B.G., Owen, D.R., & Man, F. (1993). A brief review of literature and examination of acute mood benefits of exercise in zechoslovakian and United States swimmers. *International Journal of Sport Psychology, 24,* 130-150.

Berne, E. (1964) *Games people play*. New York: Grove Press.

Berscheid, E., Walster, E., & Bohrnstedt, G. (1973, November). The happy American body. *Psychology Today*, pp. 119-131.

Biddle, S.J., & Fox, K.R. (1989). Exercise and health psychology: Emerging relationships. *British Journal of Medical Psychology, 62*, 205-216.

Blair, S.N. (1988). Exercise within a health lifestyle. In R.K. Dishman (Ed.), *Exercise adherence: Its impact on public health* (pp. 75-89). Champaign, IL: Human Kinetics.

Blaney, J., Sothman, M., Roth, H., Hart, B. & Horn, T. (1990). Impact of exercise training on plasma adrenocorticotropic response to a well-learned vigilance task. *Psychoneuroendocrinology, 15*, 453-462.

Blumenthal, J.A., Williams, R.S., Needels, T.L., & Wallace, A.G. (1982). Psychological changes accompanying aerobic exercise in healthy middle-aged adults. *Psychosomatic Medicine, 44*, 529-536.

Bolles, R.C., & Fanselow, M.S. (1982). Endorphins and behavior. In M.R. Rosenweig & L.W. Porter (Eds.), *Annual review of psychology* (Vol. 33). Palo Alto, CA: Annual Reviews Inc.

Borg, G. (1982). The rating of perceived exertion scale. *Medicine and Science in Sports and Exercise, 14*, 377-387.

Borg, G. (1985). *An introduction to Borg's RPE scale*. Ithaca, NY: Mouvement.

Bortner, R.W. (1969). A short rating scale as a potential measure of pattern A behavior. *Journal of Chronic Disease, 22*, 87-91.

Bortz, W. (1982, April). The runner's high. *Runner's World*, pp. 55-88.

Bosscher, R.J. (1993). Running and mixed physical exercises with depressed psychiatric patients. *International Journal of Sport Psychology, 24*, 170-184.

Boutcher, S.H. (1986). *The effects of running and nicotine on mood states*. Unpublished doctoral dissertation, Arizona State University, Tempe: AZ.

Boutcher, S.H., & Landers, D.M. (1988). The effects of vigorous exercise on anxiety, heart rate, and alpha activity of runners and nonrunners. *Psychophysiology, 25*, 696-702.

Brinkman, J., & Hoskins, T.A. (1979). Physical conditioning and altered self-concept in rehabilitated hemiplegic patients. *Physical Therapy, 59*, 859-865.

British Columbia Department of Health. (1978). *The PAR-Q Validation Report* (Modified Version), Gloucester, Ont.

Brown, B.S., Payne, T., Kin, C., Moore, P., & Martin, W. (1979). Chronic response of rat brain norepinephrine and serotonin levels of endurance training. *Journal of Applied Phsyiology, 46*, 19-23.

Brown, B.S., & Van Huss, W.D. (1973). Exercise and brain catecholamines. *Journal of Applied Physiology, 34*, 664-669.

Brown, D.L. (1984). The effects of exercise reconditioning on cognitive performance and affective status in patients with chronic obstructive pulmonary disease (Doctoral dissertation, University of Washington, 1983). *Dissertation Abstracts International, 45*, 662B.

Brown, D.R. (1990). Exercise, fitness, and mental health. In R. Bouchard, R. Shephard, T. Stephens, J. Sutton, & B. McPherson (Eds.), *Exercise, fitness and health* (pp. 607-626). Champaign, IL: Human Kinetics.

Brown, D.R. (1992). Physical activity, ageing, and psychological well-being: An overview of the research. *Canadian Journal of Sports Sciences, 17*, 185-193.

Brown, D.R., Morgan, W.P., & Raglin, J.S. (1993). Effects of exercise and rest on the state anxiety and blood pressure of physically challenged college students. *The Journal of Sports Medicine and Physical Fitness, 33*, 300-305.

Brown, E.Y., Morrow, J.R., & Livingston, S.M. (1982). Self-concept in women as a result of training. *Journal of Sport Psychology, 4*, 354-363.

Brown, R.S., Ramivez, D.E., & Taub, J.M. (1978). The prescription of exercise for depression. *The Physician and Sports Medicine, 6*, 34-49.

Brozek, J., & Keys, A. (1951). The evaluation of leanness-fatness in man: Norms and interrelationships. *British Journal of Nutrition, 5*, 194-206.

Brunner, B.C. (1969). Personality and motivating factors influencing adult participation in vigorous physical activity. *Research Quarterly, 40*, 464-469.

Bruya, L.D. (1977). Effect of selected movement skills on positive self-concept. *Perceptual and Motor Skills, 45*, 252-254.

Buccola, V.A., & Stone, W.J. (1975). Effects of jogging and cycling programs on physiological and personality variables in aged men. *Research Quarterly, 46*, 134-139.

Buchman, B.P., Sallis, J.F., Criqui, M.H., Dimsdale, J.E., & Kaplan, R.M. (1991). Physical activity, physical fitness, and psychological characteristics of medical students. *Journal of Psychosomatic Research, 35*, 197-208.

Bulbulian, R., & Dorabos, B.L. (1986). Motor neuron excitability: The Hoffman reflex following exercise of low and high intensity. *Medicine and Science in Sports and Exercise, 18,* 697-702.

Burgess, S.S. (1976). *Stimulus seeking, extraversion, and neuroticism in regular, occasional, and non-exercisers.* Unpublished master's thesis, Florida State University, Tallahassee.

Burns, D.D. (1980). *Feeling good: The new mood therapy.* New York: Signet Books.

Califano, J.A. (1979). *Healthy People: The Surgeon General's Report on Health Promotion and Disease Prevention* (DHEW Publication No. 79-55071). Washington, D.C.: U.S. Government Printing Office.

Cameron, O.G., & Hudson, C.J. (1986). Influence of exercise on anxiety level in patients with anxiety disorders. *Psychosomatics, 27,* 720-723.

Campbell, D.T., & Stanley, J.C. (1963). *Experimental and quasi-experimental designs for research.* Chicago: Rand McNally.

Canadian Standardized Test of Fitness (1987). *Operations manual* (3rd ed.). Ottawa: Minister of Supplies and Services Canada.

Cannon, J.G. & Kluger, M.J. (1983). Endogenous pyrogen activity in human plasma after exercise. *Science, 220,* 617-619.

Carl, J.L. (1984). The effect of aerobic exercise and group counseling on the reduction of anxiety in special education students (Doctoral dissertation, University of Southern California, 1983). *Dissertation Abstracts International, 44,* 2090A.

Carr, D.B., Bullen, B.A., Skinrar, G., Arnold, M.A., Rosenblatt, M., Beitins, I.Z., Martin, J.B., & McArthur, J.W. (1981). Physical conditioning factilitates the exercised-induced secretion of Beta-endorphin and Beta-lipotropin in women. *The New England Journal of Medicine, 305,* 560-563.

Carron, A.V. (1980). *Social psychology of sport.* Ithaca, NY: Mouvement Publications.

Caruso, C.M., Dzewaltowski, P.A., Gill, D.L. & McElroy, M.A. (1990). Psychological and physiological changes in competitive state anxiety during noncompetition and competitive success and failure. *Journal of Sport and Exercise Psychology, 12,* 6-20.

Cattell, R.B. (1956). *The 16 Personality Factor Test.* Champaign, IL: Institute for Personality and Ability Testing.

Cattell, R.B. (1965). *The scientific analysis of personality.* Baltimore: Penguin.

Cattell, R.B., & Scheier, I.H. (1958). The nature of anxiety: A review of thirteen multivariate analyses comprising 814 variables. *Psychological Reports, 4*, 351-388.

Cattell, R.B., & Scheier, I.H. (1961). *The meaning and measurement of neuroticism and anxiety.* New York: Ronald Press.

Christie, M.J., & Chesher, G.B. (1982). Physical dependence on physiologically released endogenous opiates. *Life Science, 30*, 1173-1177.

Clausen, J.P. (1977). Effect of physical training on cardiovascular adjustments to exercise in man. *Physiology Review, 57*, 779-816.

Clayton, R.P., Cox, R.H., Howley, E.T., Lawler, K.A., & Lawler, J.E. (1988). Aerobic power and cardiovascular response to stress. *Journal of Applied Physiology, 65*, 1416-1423.

Collingwood, T.R. (1972). The effects of physical training upon behavior and self-attitudes. *Journal of Clinical Psychology, 28*, 583-585.

Collingwood, T.R., & Willet, L. (1971). The effects of physical training upon self-concept and body attitude. *Journal of Clinical Psychology, 27*, 411-412.

Colt, E., Wardlaw, S., & Frantz, A.G. (1981). The effect of running on plasma B-endorphin. *Life Science, 28*, 1637.

Contrada, R.J., & Krantz, D.S. (1988). Stress reactivity and Type A behavior: Current status and future direction. *Annals of Behavioral Medicine, 10*, 64-70.

Cooper, K.G. (1968). *Aerobics.* New York: Bantam Books.

Cooper, K.G. (1977). *The aerobics way.* New York: Bantam Books.

Coopersmith, S. (1967). *The antecedents of self-esteem.* San Francisco: Freeman.

Cox, R.H. (1990). *Sport psychology: Concepts and applications.* Dubuque, IA: Wm. C. Brown.

Crandall, R. (1973). The measurement of self-esteem and related constructs. In J. Robinson & P. Shaver (Eds.), *Measures of social psychological attitude* (pp. 134-162). Ann Arbor, MI: Institute for Social Research.

Crews, D.J., & Landers, D.M. (1987). A meta-analytic review of aerobic fitness and reactivity to psychosocial stressors. *Medicine and Science in Sports and Exercise, 19*, 114-120.

Crocker, P.R., & Grozelle, C. (1991). Reducing induced state anxiety: Effects of acute aerobic exercise and autogenic relaxation. *The Journal of Sports Medicine and Physical Fitness, 31*, 277-282.

Cureton, T.K. (1963). Improvement of psychological states by means of exercise-fitness programs. *Journal of the Association for Physical and Mental Rehabilitation, 17,* 14-25.

Daniels, F.S., & Fernhall, B. (1984). Continuous EEG measurement to determine the onset of a relaxation response during a prolonged run. *Medicine and Science in Sports and Exercise, 16,* 182.

Darden, E. (1972). Sixteen personality profiles of competitive body builders and weightlifters. *Research Quarterly, 43,* 142-147.

Daugherty, P.L., Fernhall, B., & McCanne, T.R. (1987). The effects of three exercise intensities on the alpha brain wave activity of adult males. *Medicine and Science in Sports and Exercise, 19,* S23.

Davis, W.M. (1971). The effects of a cardiovascular conditioning program on selected psychological responses of colllege males (Doctoral dissertation, University of Oklahoma, 1970). *Dissertation Abstracts International, 32,* 221A.

De Geus, E.J., Lorenz, J.P., VanDoornen, L.J., & Orlebeke, J.F. (1993) Regular exercise and aerobic fitness in relation to psychosocial make-up and physiological stress reactivity. *Psychosomatic Medicine, 55,* 347-363.

Department of Health and Human Services (1980). *Promoting health/preventing disease: Objectives for the nation.* Washington DC: US Government Printing Office.

Desharnais, R., Jobin, J., Cote, C., Levesque, L., & Godin, G. (1993). Aerobic exercise and the placebo effect. *Psychsomatic Medicine, 55,* 149-154.

deVries, H.A. (1965). Effects of exercise upon residual neuromuscular tension. *Bulletin of the American Association of Electromyography, 12,* 12.

deVries, H.A. (1968). Immediate and long term effects of exercise upon resting muscle action potential. *Sports Medicine and Physical Fitness, 8,* 1-11.

deVries, H.A. (1981). Tranquilizer effect of exercise: A critical review. *The Physician and Sportsmedicine, 9,* 46-55.

deVries, H.A., Beckman, P., Huber, H., & Dieckmeir, L. (1968). Electromyographic evaluation of the effects of sauna on the neuromuscular system. *Journal of Sports Medicine and Physical Fitness, 8,* 1-11.

deVries, H.A., Simard, C.P., & Wiswell, R.A. (1982). Fusimotor system involvement in the tranquilizer effect of exercise. *American Journal of Physical Medicine, 61,* 111-122.

deVries, H.A., Wiswell, R.A., Bulbulian, R., & Moritani, T.(1981). Tranquilizer effect of exercise. *American Journal of Physical Medicine, 60,* 57-66.

DiClemente, C.C. (1981). Self-efficacy and smoking cessation maintenance: A preliminary report. *Cognitive Therapy Research, 5,* 175-187.

Dienstbier, R.A. (1984). The effects of exercise on personality. In M. Sachs & G. Buffone (Eds.), *Running as therapy: An integrated approach* (pp. 253-272. Lincoln NA: University of Nebraska.

Dienstbier, R.A. (1984). Arousal and physiological toughness: Implications for mental and physical health. *Psychological Review, 96,* 84-100.

Dienstbier, R.A., Crabbe, J., & Johnson, G.U. (1981). Exercise and stress tolerance. In M.H. Sacks, & M.L Sachs (Eds.), *Psychology of running* (pp. 192-210). Champaign, IL: Human Kinetics.

Dishman, R.K. (1982). Contemporary sport psychology. In R.L. Terjung (Ed.), *Exercise and Sport Science Reviews, 10,* 120-159.

Dishman, R.K. (1985). Medical psychology in exercise and sport. *Medical Clinics of North America, 69,* 123-143.

Dishman, R.K. (1986). Mental health. In V. Seefeldt (Ed.), *Physical activity and well-being* (pp. 304-340). Reston, VA: American Association for Health, Physical Education and Recreation Publications.

Dishman, R.K. (1994). Biological psychology, exercise, and stress. *Quest, 46,* 28-59.

Dishman, R.K., Sallis, J.F., & Orenstein, D.R. (1985). The determinants of physical activity and exercise. *Public Health Reports, 100,* 158-171.

Doan, R.E., & Scherman, A. (1987). The therapeutic effect of physical fitness on measures of personality: A literature review. *Journal of Counseling and Development, 66,* 28-36.

Doctor, R., & Sharkey, B.J. (1971). Note on some physiological and subjective reactions to exercise and training. *Perceptual and Motor Skills, 32,* 233-237.

Douchamps-Riboux, F., Heinz, J.K., & Douchamps, J. (1989) Arousal as a tridimensional variable: An exploratory study of behavior changes in rowers following a marathon race. *International Journal of Sport Psychology, 20,* 31-41.

Doyne, E.J., Chambless, D.L., & Beutler, L.E. (1983). Aerobic exercise as a treatment for depression in women. *Behavior Therapy, 14,* 434-440.

Doyne, E.J., Ossip-Klein, D.J., Bowman, E.D., Osborn, K.M., McDougall-Wilson, J.B., & Neimeyer, R.A. (1987). Running versus weight lifting in the treatment of depression. *Journal of Consulting and Clinical Psychology, 55,* 748-754.

Driscoll, R. (1976). Anxiety reduction using physical exertion and positive images. *Psychological Record, 26,* 87-94.

Dunn, A.L., & Dishman, R.K. (1991). Exercise and the neurobiology of depression. *Exercise and Sport Sciences Reviews, 19,* 41-98.

Durden-Smith, J. (1978). A chemical cure for madness. *Quest, 2,* 31-36.

Dyer, J.B., & Crouch, J.G. (1987). Effects of running on moods:A time series study. *Perceptual and Motor Skills, 64,* 783-789.

Dyer, J.B., & Crouch, J.G. (1988). Effects of running and other activities on moods. *Perceptual and Motor Skills, 67,* 43-50.

Eby, J.M. (1985). An investigation into the effects of aerobic exercise on anxiety and depression (Doctoral dissertation, University of Toronto, 1984). *Dissertation Abstracts International, 46,* 1734B.

Eichman, W.J. (1978). Profile of mood states. In O.K. Buros (Ed.), *The eighth mental measurements yearbook* (pp. 1016-1018). Highland Park,NJ: Gryphon Press.

Emery, C.F. (1986). The effect of physical exercise on cognitive and psychological functioning in community aged (Doctoral dissertation, University of Southern California, 1985). *Dissertation Abstracts International, 46,* 4384B.

Emery, C.F., & Gatz, M. (1990). Psychological and cognitive effects of an exercise program for community-residing older adults. *The Gerontologist, 30,* 184-188.

Endler, N.S., & Hunt, J.M. (1966). Sources of behavior variance as measured by the S-R Inventory of Anxiousness. *Psychological Bulletin, 65,* 338-346.

Endler, N.S., & Hunt, J.M. (1968). Inventories of hostility and comparisons of the proportions of variance from persons, responses, and situations for hostility and anxiousness. *Journal of Personality and Social Psychology, 9,* 309-315.

Ewart, C.K., Taylor, C.B., Reise, L.B., & DeBusk, R.F. (1983). Effects of early postmyocardial infarction exercise testing on self-perception and subsequent physical activity. *American Journal of Cardiology, 51,* 1076-1080.

Eysenck, H. (1960). *The structure of human personality.* London: Methuen.

Fardy, P.S., Yanowotz, F.G., & Wilson, P.K. (1988). *Cardiac rehabilitation, adult fitness, and exercise testing.* Philadelphia: Lea & Febiger.

Farmer, P.K., Olewine, D.A., & Comer, D.W. (1978). Frontalis muscle tension and occipital alpha production in young males with coronary prone (type A) and coronary resistant (type B) behavior patterns. *Medicine and Science in Sports and Exercise, 10,* 51.

Farrell, P.A. (1989). Lack of exercise effects on peripheral enkephalin entry into whole brain of rats. *Medicine and Science in Sports and Exercise, 21,* S35.

Federici, J.R. (1986). The effect of regular exercise on depressive symptomology (Doctoral dissertation, United States International University, 1985). *Dissertation Abstracts International, 47,* 2613B.

Fehr, F.S., & Stern, J.A. (1970). Peripheral physiological variables and emotion: The James-Lange theory revisited. *Psychological Bulletin, 74,* 411-424.

Felts, W.M. (1984). Effects of acute exercise on postexercise arousal, stress reactivity, and state anxiety as a function of aerobic fitness level (Doctoral dissertation, University of Maryland, 1983). *Dissertation Abstracts International, 44,* 2986A.

Felts, W.M. (1989). Relationship between ratings of perceived exertion and exercise-induced decreases in state anxiety. *Perceptual and Motor Skills, 69,* 368-370.

Fenichel, O. (1954). *Collected papers of Otto Fenichel* (1st ed.). New York: Norton.

Fernhall, B., & Daniels, F.S. (1984). Electroencephalographic changes after a prolonged running period: Evidence for a relaxation response. *Medicine and Science in Sports and Exercise, 16,* 181.

Festinger, L. (1957). *A theory of cognitive dissonance.* Stanford, CA: Stanford University Press.

Fieve, R.R. (1989). *Moodswing.* New York:Bantam Books.

Fisher, A.C. (1984). New directions in personality research. In J. Silva & R. Weinberg (Eds.), *Psychological foundations in sport* (pp. 70-80). Champaign IL: Human Kinetics.

Fisher, S., & Cleveland, S.E. (1968). *Body image and personality.* New York: Dover.

Fitness Canada (1986). *Canada fitness survey - highlights* Ottawa: Government of Canada.

Fitts, W.H. (1964). *Tennessee Self-Concept Scale.* Nashville, TN: Counselor Recordings and Tests.

Flory, J.D., & Holmes, D.S. (1991). Effects of an acute bout of aerobic exercise on cardiovascular and subjective responses during subsequent cognitive work. *Journal of Psychosomatic Research, 35,* 225-230.

Folkins, C.H. (1976). Effects of physical training on mood. *Journal of Clinical Psychology, 32,* 385-388.

Folkins, C.H., Lynch, S., & Gardner, M.M. (1972). Psychological fitness as a function of physical fitness. *Archives of Physical Medicine and Rehabilitation, 53,* 503-508.

Folkins, C.H., & Sime, W.F. (1981). Physical fitness training and mental health. *American Psychologist, 35,* 373-389.

Ford, H.T., Puckett, J.R., Blessing, D.L., & Tucker, L.A. (1989). Effects of selected physical activities on health-related fitness and psychological well-being. *Psychological Reports, 64,* 203-208.

Fourman, J.L. (1989). The effects of exercise on anxiety in pregnant women (Doctoral dissertation, University of Western Michigan, 1988). *Dissertation Abstracts International, 49,* 2913B.

Fox, S.M., & Haskell, W.L. (1978). Physical activity and the prevention of coronary heart disease. *New York Academy Medical Bulletin, 53,* 950-965.

Franz, S.I., & Hamilton, G.V. (1905). The effects of exercise upon the retardation in conditions of depression. *American Journal of Insanity, 62,* 239-256.

Frazier, S.E., & Nagy, S. (1989). Mood state changes of women as a function of regular aerobic exercise. *Perceptual and Motor Skills, 68,* 283-287.

Frederick, C.M., & Ryan, R.M. (1993). Differences in motivation for sport and exercise and their relations with participation and mental health. *Journal of Sport Behavior, 16,* 124-126.

Fremont, J. (1984). The separate and combined effects of cognitive based counseling and aerobic exercise for the treatment of mild and moderate depression (Doctoral dissertation, Penn State University, 1983) *Dissertation Abstracts International, 44,* 2413A.

Fremont, J., & Craighead, L.W. (1987). Aerobic exercise and cognitive therapy in the treatment of dysphoric moods. *Cognitive Therapy and Research, 11,* 241-251.

Freud, S. (1900). *The interpretation of dreams.* In standard edition, Vols. 4 & 5, London: Hogarth Press, 1953.

Freud, S. (1901). *The psychopathology of everyday life.* In standard edition, Vol. 6, London:Hogarth Press, 1960.

Freud, S. (1917). *Introductory lectures on psychoanalysis.* In standard edition, Vols. 15 & 16, London: Hogarth Press, 1963.

Freud, S. (1963). *The problem of anxiety.* New York: Psychoanalytic Quarterly Press.

Friday, W.W. (1987). Physiological, psychological, and behavioral effects of aerobic exercise and cognitive experiential therapy on juvenile delinquent males (Doctoral dissertation, Ohio State University, 1987). *Dissertation Abstracts International, 48,* 1707A.

Fromm, E. (1956). *The art of loving.* New York: Harper & Row.

Garver, D.L., & Davis, J.M. (1979). Minireview: Biogenic amine hypotheses of affective disorders. *Life Sciences, 24,* 383-394.

Gary, V., & Gutherie, D. (1972). The effect of jogging on physical fitness and self-concept in hospitalized alcoholics. *Quarterly Journal of Studies on Alcohol, 33,* 1073-1078.

Gauvin, L. (1989). The relationship between regular physical activity and subjective well-being. *Journal of Sport Behavior, 12,* 107-114.

Gergen, K.J. (1971). *The concept of self.* New York: Holt.

Glass, G.V. (1976). Primary, secondary, and meta-analysis of research. *Education Research, 5,* 3-8.

Glass, G.V., McGaw, B., & Smith, M.L. (1981). *Meta-analysis in social research.* Beverly Hills, CA: Sage Publications.

Glasser, W. (1976). *Positive addiction.* New York: Harper & Row.

Gleser, J., & Mendelberg, H. (1990). Exercise and sport in mental health: A review of the literature. *Israel Journal of Psychiatry and Related Science, 27,* 99-112.

Goldstein, W.N., & Anthony, R.N. (1988). The diagnosis of depression and the DSM's. *American Journal of Psychotherapy, 42,* 180-196.

Goldwater, B.C., & Collis, M.L. (1985). Psychologic effects of cardiovascular conditioning: A controlled experiment. *Psychosomatic Medicine, 47,* 174-181.

Goode, D.J., Dekirmenjian, H., Meltzer, H.Y., & Maas, J.W. (1973). Relation of exercise to MHPG excretion in normal subjects. *Archives of General Psychiatry, 29,* 391-396.

Goodman, J. (1992). Assessment of exercise capacity and principles of exercise prescription. In R.J. Shephard and H.S. Miller (Eds.), *Exercise and the heart in health and disease* (pp. 55-103). New York: Marcel Dekker, Inc.

Goodman, J.M., & Goodman, L.S. (1985). Exercise prescription for the sedentary adult. In R.P. Welsh, & R.J. Shephard (Eds.), *Current therapy in sports medicine*. Philadelphia: B.G. Decker.

Greenwood, C.M., Dzewaltowski, D.A., & French, R. (1990). Self-efficacy and psychological well-being of wheelchair tennis participants and wheelchair nontennis participants. *Adapted Physical Activity Quarterly, 7*, 12-21.

Greist, J.H. (1987). Exercise intervention with depressed outpatients. In W. Morgan & S. Goldston (Eds), *Exercise and mental health* (pp. 117-121). Washington DC: Hemisphere Publishers.

Greist, J.H., Klein, M.H., Eischens, R.R., Faris, J., Gurman, A.S., & Morgan, W.P. (1979). Running as treatment for depression. *Comprehensive Psychiatry, 20*, 41-54.

Griffith, J.S. (1984). Exercise as a coping resource in reducing anxiety and mediating stressful life events (Doctoral dissertation, University of Pittsburgh, 1983). *Dissertation Abstracts International, 44*, 2360A.

Gussis, L. (1971). The influence of selected sport skills-oriented programs on the self-concept of body-image of boys in grade ten (Doctoral dissertation, Boston University, 1971). *Dissertation Abstracts International, 32*, 1902A.

Haier, R.J., Quaid, B.A., & Mills, J.S. (1981). Naloxone alters pain perception after jogging [letter]. *Psychiatry Research, 5*, 231-232.

Haight, J.S., & Keatinge, W.R. (1973). Elevation in set point for body temperature regulation after prolonged exercise. *Journal of Physiology, 229*, 77-85.

Hamachek, D.E. (1986). Enhancing the self's psychology by improving fitness physiology. *Journal of Human Behavior and Learning, 3*, 2-12.

Hamachek, D.E. (1987). *Encounters with the self* (3rd ed.). New York: Holt, Rinehart, & Winston.

Hammer, W.M., & Wilmore, J.H. (1973). An exploratory investigation in personality measures and physiological alterations during a 10-week jogging program. *Journal of Sports Medicine and Physical Fitness, 13*, 238-247.

Hannaford, C.P., Harrell, E.H., & Cox, K. (1988). Psychophysiological effects of a running program on depression and anxiety in a psychiatric population. *The Psychological Record, 38*, 37-48.

Hannum, S.M., & Kasch, F.W. (1981). Acute post exercise blood pressure response of hypertensive and normotensive men. *Scandanavian Journal of Sports Science, 3*, 1, 11-15.

Hanson, J.S., & Nedde, W.H. (1974). Long term physical training effect in sedentary females. *Journal of Applied Physiology, 37*, 112-116.

Hardy, C.J., & Rejeski, W.J. (1989). Not what, but how one feels: The measurement of affect during exercise. *Journal of Sport and Exercise Psychology, 11*, 304-317.

Harris, D.V. (1966). An investigation of psychological characteristics of university women with high and low fitness (Doctoral dissertation, University of Iowa, 1965). *Dissertation Abstracts International, 26*, 5851.

Harris, D.V. (1978, Jan.). The happy addict. *Womensports, 5*, 53.

Harris, L. (1979). *The Perrier study: Fitness in America.* New York: Great Waters of France.

Harter, S. (1978). Effectance motivation reconsidered: Toward a   developmental model. *Human Development, 21*, 34-64.

Hartley, L.H., Mason, J.W., Hogan, R.P., Jones, L.G., Kotchen, T.A., Mougey, E.H., Wherry, F.E., Pennington, L.L., & Ricketts, P.T. (1972). Multiple hormonal response to graded exercise in relatin to physical training. *Journal of Applied Physiology, 33*, 602-606.

Hartung, G.H., & Farge, E.J. (1977). Personality and physiological traits in middle-aged runners and joggers. *Journal of Gerontology, 32*, 541-548.

Hathaway, S.R., & McKinley, J.C. (1943). *Minnesota Multiphasic Personality Inventory: Manual.* New York: Psychological Corporation.

Hayden, R.M., & Allen, C.J. (1984). Relationships between aerobic exercise, anxiety, and depression: Convergent validation by knowledgeable informants. *Journal of Sports Medicine, 24*, 68-74.

Health and Welfare Canada. (1988). *The body mass index.* Ottawa: Expert Group on Weight Standards.

Heinzelman, I., & Bagley, R.W. (1970). Response to physical activity programs and their effects on health behavior. *Public Health Reports, 85*, 905-911.

Hellison, D.R. (1970). The effect of physical conditioning on affective attitudes toward the self, the body and physical fitness (Doctoral dissertation, United States International Univesity, 1969). *Dissertation Abstracts International, 30*, 2831A.

Henderson, J. (1974). The effect of physical conditioning on self-concept in college women (Doctoral dissertation, Washington State University, 1974). *Dissertation Abstracts International, 35*, 3063B.

Henning, J.M. (1987). The effects of a regular exercise program on the self-concept and self-actualization of geriatric patients (Doctoral dissertation,

United States International University, 1987). *Dissertation Abstracts International, 48,* 1800B.

Hersen, M., & Barlow, D. (1976). *Single case experimental designs: Strategies for studying behavior change.* New York: Pergamon Press.

Hill, S.D. (1968). Depression: disease, reaction or posture. *American Journal of Psychology, 125,* 445-457.

Hilyer, J.D., & Mitchell, J.W. (1979). Effect of systematic physical fitness training combined with counseling on the self-concept of college students. *Journal of Counseling Psychology, 26,* 427-436.

Hogan, J. (1989). Personality correlates of physical fitness. *Journal of Personality and Social Psychology, 56,* 284-288.

Hogan, R. (1986). *Hogan Personality Inventory manual.* Minneapolis, MN: National Computer Systems.

Holland, R.L., Sayers, J.A., Keatinge, W.R., Davis, H.M., & Pestwani, R. (1985). Effects of raised body temperature on reasoning, memory, and mood. *Journal of Applied Physiology, 59,* 1823-1827.

Holloszy, J.O. (1983). Exercise, health, and aging: A need for more information. *Medicine and Science in Sports and Exercise, 15,* 1-5.

Holmes, D.S., & Roth, D.L. (1985). Association of aerobic fitness with pulse rate and subjective responses to psychological stress. *Psychophysiology, 22,* 525-529.

Horne, J.A., & Staff, C.H. (1983). Exercise and sleep: Body heating effects. *Sleep, 6,* 36-46.

Horney, K. (1950). *Neurosis and human growth.* New York: Morton.

Horney, K. (1924). On the genesis of the castration complex in women. *International Journal of Psychoanalysis, 5,* 50-65.

Howlett, D.R. , & Jenner, F.A. (1978). Studies relating to the clinical significance of urinary 3-methoxy-4-hydroxyphenylethylene glycol. *British Journal of Psychiatry, 132,* 49-54.

Howley, E.T. (1981). The excretion of catecholamines as an index of exercise stress. In F.J. Nagel & H.J. Montoye (Eds.), *Exercise in health and disease* (pp. 22-31). Springfield, IL: Charles C. Thomas.

Howley, E.T., & Franks, B.D. (1986). *Health/fitness instructor's handbook.* Champaign, IL: Human Kinetics Pub.

Hughes, J., Smith, T.W., Kosterlitz, H.W., Fothergill, L.A., Morgan, B.A., & Morris, H.R. (1975). Identification of two related pentapeptides from the brain with potent opiate agonist activity. *Nature, 258,* 577-579.

Hughes, J.R. (1984). Psychological effects of habitual aerobic exercise: A critical review. *Preventive Medicine, 13*, 66-78.

Hughes, J.R., Casal, D.C., & Leon, A.S. (1986). Psychological effects of exercise: A randomized cross-over trial. *Journal of Psychosomatic Research, 30*, 355-360.

Hull, E.M., Young, S.H., & Zeigler, M.G. (1984). Aerobic fitness affects cardiovascular and catecholamine responses to stressors. *Psychophysiology, 21*, 353-360.

Illich, I. (1976). *Limits to medicine*. New York: Penguin Books.

Ismail, A.H., & Trachtman, L.E. (1973). Jogging the imagination. *Psychology Today*, pp. 78-82.

Ismail, A.H., & Young, R.J. (1977). Effect of chronic exercise on the personality of adults. *Annals of the New York Academy of Science, 301*, 959-969.

Jackson, A., Watkins, M., & Patton, R. (1980). A factor analysis of twelve selected maximal isotonic strength performances on the Universal Gym. *Medicine and Science in Sports and Exercise, 12*, 274-277.

Jasnoski, M., & Holmes, D.S. (1981). Influence of initial aerobic fitness, aerobic training, and changes in aerobic fitness on personality functioning. *Journal of Psychosomatic Research, 25*, 553-556.

Jasnoski, M., Holmes, D.S., & Banks, D.L. (1988). Changes in personality associated with changes in aerobic and anaerobic fitness in women and men. *Journal of Psychosomatic Research, 32*, 273-276.

Jasnoski, M.L., Holmes, D.S., Soleman, S., & Agular, C. (1981). Exercise, changes in aerobic capacity, and changes in self-perceptions: An experimental investigation. *Journal of Research in Personality, 15*, 460-466.

Jeffers, J. (1977). The effects of physical conditioning on locus of control, body image and interpersonal relationship orientation of university males and females (Doctoral dissertation, East Texas State University, 1977). *Dissertation Abstracts International, 38*, 3289A.

Jewell, R. (1987). Aerobic exercise: Strength of relationships between fitness changes and psychological changes, a repeated measures approach (Doctoral dissertation, Brigham Young University, 1987). *Dissertation Abstracts International, 48*, 878B.

Jin, P. (1989). Changes in heart rate, noradrenaline, cortisol, and mood during TaiChi. *Journal of Psychosomatic Research, 3*, 197-206.

Joesting, G., & Clance, P. (1979). Comparison of runners and nonrunners on the body-cathexis and self-cathexis scales. *Perceptual and Motor Skills, 48*, 1046.

Johnsgard, K.W. (1989). *The exercise prescription for anxiety and depression.* New York: Plenum Publishing.

Johnson, J.A. (1986). The effects of group and individual running therapy on depression (Doctoral dissertation, University of Arkansas, 1985). *Dissertation Abstracts International, 46,* 2926B.

Johnston, B. (1970). A study of the relationships among self-concept, movement concept and physical fitness and the effects of a physical conditioning program upon self-concept and movement concept (Doctoral dissertation, Florida State University, 1969). *Dissertation Abstracts International, 30,* 5270A-5271A.

Jones, R.D., & Weinhouse, S. (1979). Running as selftherapy. *Journal of Sports Medicine, 19,* 397-404.

Jung, C.G. (1926). The structure and dynamics of the psyche. In *Collected Works* (Vol. 8). Princeton: University Press.

Kahle, L.R., Kulka, R.A., & Klinger, D.M. (1980). Low adolescent self-esteem leads to multiple interpersonal problems: A test of social-adaptation theory. *Journal of Personality and Social Psychology, 39,* 496-502.

Kamman, R., & Flett, R. (1983). Measure of current level of general happiness. *Australian Journal of Psychiatry, 35,* 259-265.

Kamp, A., & Troost, J. (1978). EEG signs of cerebrovascular disorder, using physical exercise as a provocative method. *Electroencephalography and Clinical Neurophysiology, 45,* 295-298.

Katz, J.L. (1986). Long distance running, anorexia nervosa, and bulimia: A report of two case studies. *Comprehensive Psychiatry, 27,* 74-78.

Kavanaugh, T., Shephard, R.J., Tuck, J.A., & Qureshi, S. (1977). Depression following myocardial infarction: The effects of distance running. *Annals of the New York Academy of Science, 801,* 1029-1036.

Keller, S., & Seraganian, P. (1984). Physical fitness level and autonomic reactivity in psychosocial stress. *Journal of Psychosomatic Research, 28,* 279-287.

Kendall, P.C., & Branswell, L. (1982). Cognitive behavioral self-control therapy for children: A components analysis. *Journal of Consulting and Clinical Psychology, 50,* 672-689.

Kerr, J.H., & Vlaswinkel, E.H. (1990). Effects of exercise on anxiety: A review. *Anxiety Research, 2,* 309-321.

King, A., Barr Taylor, C., & Haskell, W.L. (1993). Effects of differing intensities and formats of 12 months of exercise training on psychological outcomes in older adults. *Health Psychology, 12,* 292-300.

King, A., Barr Taylor, C., Haskell, W.L., & DeBusk, R.F. (1989). Influence of regular exercise on psychological health: A randomized controlled trial of healthy middle-aged adults. *Health Psychology, 8*, 305-324.

Kirkcaldy, B.D., & Shephard, R.J. (1990). Therapeutic implications of exercise. *International Journal of Sport Psychology, 21*, 165-184.

Klein, M. (1950). *The psychoanalysis of children.* London: Hogarth Press.

Klein, M.H., Greist, J.H., Gurman, A.S., Neimeyer, R.A., Lesser, D.P., Bushnell, N.J., & Smith, R.E. (1985). A comparative outcome study of group psychotherapy vs. exercise treatments for depression. *International Journal of Mental Health, 13*, 148-177.

Kostrabula, T. (1976). *The joy of running.* Philadelphia: J.B. Lippincott.

Kostrabula, T. (1981). Running and psychotherapy. In S.I Fuenning, K.D. Rose, F.D. Strider, & W.E. Sime (Eds.), *Physical fitness and mental health: Proceedings of the research seminar on physical fitness and mental health.* Lincoln, NE: University of Nebraska Foundation.

Kowal, D.M., Payton, J.F., & Vogel, J.A. (1978). Psychological states and aerobic fitness of male and female recruits before and after basic training. *Aviation, Space, and Environmental Medicine, 49*, 603-608.

Kugler, J., Dimsdale, J., Hartley, L., & Sherwood, J. (1990). Hospital supervised vs. home exercise in cardiac rehabilitation: Effects on aerobic fitness, anxiety, and depression. *Archives of Physical Medicine Rehabilitation, 71*, 322-325.

Kuhn, T.S. (1970). *The structure of scientific revolutions* (2nd ed.). Chicago: Univesity of Chicago Press.

Kuyler, P.L., & Dunner, D.L. (1976). Psychiatric disorders and the need for mental health services among a sample of orthopedic inpatients. *Comprehensive Psychiatry, 17*, 395-400.

Labbe, E.E., Welsh, M.C., & Delaney, D. (1988). Effects of consistent aerobic exercise on the psychological functioning of women. *Perceptual and Motor Skills, 67*, 919-925.

Lake, B.W., Suarex, E.C., Schneiderman, N., & Tocci, N. (1985). The type A behavior pattern, physical fitness, and psychological reactivity. *Health Psychology, 4*, 169-187.

Landers, D.M. (1994). Performance, stress, and health: Overall reaction. *Quest, 46*, 123-135.

Layman, E.M. (1960). Contributions of exercise and sports to mental health and social adjustment. In W.R. Johnson (Ed.), *Science and medicine in exercise and sports* (pp. 560-599). New York: Harper and Brothers.

Layman, E.M. (1972). The contributions of play and sport to emotional health. In J.E. Kane (Ed.), *Psychological aspects of physical education and sport* (pp. 163-186). London: Routledge & Kegan Paul.

Layman, E.M. (1974). Psychological effects of physical activity. In J.H. Wilmore (Ed.), *Exercise and sports sciences reviews* (pp. 33-70). New York: Academic Press.

Ledwidge, B. (1980) Run for your mind: Aerobic exercise as a means of alleviating anxiety and depression. *Canadian Journal of Behavioural Science, 12,* 126-140.

Leighton, J. (1955). An instrument and technique for the measurement of range of joint motion. *Archives of Physical Medicine and Rehabilitation, 36,* 571-578.

Leith, L.M. (1982). Psychological aspects of physical activity and aging. *Recreation Research Review, 9,* 16-22.

Leith, L.M., & Taylor, A.H. (1990). Psychological aspects of exercise: A decade literature review. *Journal of Sport Behavior, 13,* 1-22.

Leith, L.M., & Taylor, A.H. (1992). Behavior modification and exercise adherence: A literature review. *Journal of Sport Behavior, 16,* 1-15.

Lennox, S.S. (1989). The effect of aerobic exercise on self-reported mood (Doctoral dissertation, State University of New York at Stony Brook, 1987). *Dissertation Abstracts International, 49,* 3447B.

Lennox, S.S., Bedell, J.R., & Stone, A.A. (1990). The effect of exercise on normal mood. *Journal of Psychosomatic Research, 34,* 629-636.

Leonardson, G., & Garguilo, R. (1978). Self-perception and physical fitness. *Perceptual and Motor Skills, 46,* 338.

Levenkron, J.C., & Moore, L.G. (1988). The type A behavior pattern: Issues for intervention research. *Annals of Behavioral Medicine, 10,* 78-83.

Lichtman, S., & Poster, E.G. (1983). The effects of exercise on mood and cognitive functioning. *Journal of Psychosomatic Research, 27,* 43-52.

Liebert, R.M., & Morris, L.W. (1967). Cognitive and emotional components of test anxiety: A distinction and some initial data. *Psychological Reports, 20,* 975-978.

Lifton, R.D., & Nannis, E.D. (1988). Hogan Personality Inventory/Hogan Personnel Selection Series. *Test Critiques, 4,* 216-225.

Lion, L.S. (1978). Psychological effects of jogging: A preliminary study. *Perceptual and Motor Skills, 47,* 1215-1218.

Lobitz, W.C., Brammell, H.L., & Stoll, S. (1983). Physical exercise and anxiety management training for cardiac stress management in a non-patient population. *Journal of Cardiac Rehabilitation, 3*, 683-688.

Lobstein, D.D., Mosbacher, B.J., & Ismail, A.H. (1983). Depression as a powerful discriminator between physically active and sedentary middle-aged men. *Journal of Psychosomatic Research, 27*, 69-76.

Long, B. (1984). Aerobic conditioning and stress inoculation: A comparison of stress management interventions. *Cognitive Therapy and Research, 8*, 517-542.

Long, B. (1985). Stress-management interventions: A 15-month follow-up of aerobic conditioning and stress inoculation training. *Cognitive Therapy and Research, 9*, 471-478.

Long, B.C., & Haney, C.J. (1988a). Coping strategies for working women: Aerobic exercise and relaxation interventions. *Behavior Therapy, 19*, 75-83.

Long, B.C., & Haney, C.J. (1988b). Long term follow-up of stressed working women: A comparison of aerobic exercise and progressive relaxation. *Journal of Sport and Exercise Psychology, 10*, 461-470.

Long, J.W. (1991). *The essential guide to prescription drugs.* New York: Harper Collins.

Madden, M.E. (1990). Attributions of control and vulnerability at the beginning and end of a karate class. *Perceptual and Motor Skills, 70*, 787-794.

Maddi, S.R. (1984). Personology for the 1980's. In R.A. Zucker, J. Aronoff, & A.I. Rabin (Eds.), *Personality and the prediction of behavior* (pp. 7-41). Orlando, FL: Academic Press.

Maroulakis, E., & Zervas, Y. (1993). Effects of aerobic exercise on mood of adult women. *Perceptual and Motor Skills, 76*, 795-801.

Marsh, H.W. (1987). The hierarchical structure of self-concept and the application of hierarchical confirmatory factor analysis. *Journal of Educational Measurement, 24*, 17-37.

Marsh, H.W., Barnes, J., Cairns, L., & Tidman, M. (1984). The Self-Description Questionnaire (SDQ): Age effects in the structure and level of self-concept for preadolescent children. *Journal of Educational Psychology, 76*, 940-956.

Marsh, H.W., & Peart, N.D. (1988). Competitive and co-operative physical fitness training programs for girls: Effects on physical fitness and multidimensional self-concepts. *Journal of Sport and Exercise Psychology, 10*, 390-407.

Martens, R. (1975). The paradigmatic crisis in American sport personology. *Sporswissenschaft, 5,* 9-24.

Martens, R., Burton, D., Vealey, R.S., Bump, L., & Smith, D.E. (1983). *The development of the competitive state anxiety inventory - 2 (CSAI-2).* Unpublished manuscript.

Martin, C.C. (1987). Exercise as a therapeutic intervention for improving self-esteem in women: The psychological masculinity factor (Doctoral dissertation, Memphis State University, 1986). *Dissertation Abstracts International, 47,* 4306/7B.

Martin, J.E., & Dubbert, P.M. (1982). Exercise applications and promotion in behavioral medicine: Current status and future directions. *Journal of Consulting and Clinical Psychology, 50,* 1004-1017.

Martinek, T.J., Cheffers, J.T., & Zaichowsky, L.D. (1978). Physical activity, motor development, self-concept; Race and age differences. *Perceptual and Motor Skills, 26,* 147-154.

Martinsen, E.W. (1987). Exercise and medication in the psychiatric patient. In W. Morgan & S. Goldston (Eds.), *Exercise and mental health* (pp. 85-95). Washington DC: Hemisphere.

Martinsen, E.W. (1990). Physical fitness, anxiety, and depression. *British Journal of Hospital Medicine, 43,* 197-199.

Martinsen, E.W. (1993). Therapeutic implications of exercise for clinically anxious and depressed patients. *International Journal of Sport Psychology, 24,* 185-189.

Martinsen, E.W., Hoffart, A., & Solberg, O. (1989a). Aerobic and nonaerobic forms of exercise in the treatment of anxiety disorders. *Stress Medicine, 5,* 115-120.

Martinsen, E.W., Hoffart, A., & Solberg, O. (1989b). Comparing aerobic with nonaerobic forms of exercise in the treatment of clinical depression: A randomized trial. *Comprehensive Psychiatry, 30,* 324-331.

Martinsen, E.W., & Medhus, A. (1989). Adherence to exercise and patients' evaluation of physical exercise in a comprehensive treatment programme for depression. *Nordisk-Psykiatrisk-Tidsskrift, 43,* 411-415.

Martinsen, E.W., Medhus, A., & Sandvik, L. (1985). Effects of aerobic exercise on depression: A controlled study. *British Medical Journal, 291,* 109.

Mathews, A. (1978). Fear reduction research and clinical phobias. *Psychological Bulletin, 85,* 390-404.

Mauser, H. & Reynolds, R.P. (1977). Effects of a developmental physical activity program on children's body coordination and self-concept. *Perceptual and Motor Skills, 44,* 1057-1058.

May, R. (1977). *The meaning of anxiety.* New York: W.W. Norton.

Mayo, F.M. (1975). The effects of aerobics conditioning exercises on selected personality characteristics of seventh- and eigth-grade girls (Doctoral dissertation, North Texas State University, 1974). *Dissertation Abstracts International, 35,* 4162A.

McCann, I.L., & Holmes, D.S. (1984). Influence of aerobic exercise on depression. *Journal of Personality and Social Psychology, 46,* 1142-1147.

McGilley, B.M. (1987). Influence of exercise rehabilitation on coronary patients: A 6-year follow-up evaluation (Doctoral dissertation, University of Kansas, 1987). *Dissertation Abstracts International, 49,* 2382B.

McGlenn, L. (1976). Relationship of personality and self-image change on high and low fitness adolescent males to selected activity programs (Doctoral dissertation, United States International University, 1976). *Dissertation Abstracts International, 37,* 1410B-1411B.

McGowan, R.W., Jarman, G.O., & Pederson, D.M. (1974). Effects of a competitive endurance training program on self-concept and peer approval. *Journal of Psychology, 86,* 57-60.

McGowan, R.W., Pierce, E.F., Eastman, N., Tripathi, H.L., Dewey, T., & Olson, K. (1993). Beta-endorphins and mood states during resistance exercise. *Perceptual and Motor Skills, 76,* 376-378.

McGowan, R.W., Pierce, E.F., & Jordan, D. (1991). Mood alterations with a single bout of exercise. *Perceptual and Motor Skills, 72,* 1203-1209.

McIntyre, C.W., Watson, D., & Cunningham, A.C. (1990). The effects of social interaction, exercise, and test stress on positive and negative affect. *Bulletin of the Psychonomic Society, 28,* 141-143.

McNair, D.M., Lorr, N., & Droppleman, L.F. (1971). *Manual for the profile of mood states.* San Diego: Education and Industrial Testing Service.

Mead, G.W. (1934). *Mind, self, and society.* Chicago: University of Chicago Press.

Meichenbaum, D. (1977). *Cognitive behavior modification.* New York: Plenum Press.

Messer, B., & Harter, S. (1986). *Manual for the Adult Self-Perception Profile.* Denver: University of Denver.

Meyer, R., & Smith, S. (1977). A crisis in group therapy. *American Psychologist, 32,* 638-643.

Meyer, R.G., & Salmon, P. (1984). *Abnormal psychology.* Boston:Allyn & Bacon.

Millon, T. (1981). *Disorders of personality, DSM-III: Axis II.* New York: John Wiley Pub.

Mischel, W. (1968). *Personality and assessment.* New York: John Wiley Pub.

Mischel, W. (1973). Toward a cognitive social learning reconceptualization of personality. *Psychological Review, 80,* 252-283.

Mischel, W. (1977). On the future of personality measurement. *American Psychologist, 32,* 246-254.

Montgomery, S.A., & Asberg, M. (1979). A new depression scale designed to be sensitive to change. *British Journal of Psychiatry, 134,* 382-389.

Moore, M. (1982). Endorphins and exercise: A puzzling relationship. *The Physician and Sportsmedicine, 10,* 111-114.

Morgan, W.P. (1969). Physical fitness and emotional health: A review. *American Corrective Therapy Journal, 23,* 124-127.

Morgan, W.P. (1973). Efficacy of psychobiologic inquiry in the exercise and sport sciences. *Quest, 20,* 39-47.

Morgan, W.P. (1974). Exercise and mental disorders. In A.J. Ryan, & F.L. Allman (Eds.), *Sports medicine* (pp. 671-678). New York: Academic Press.

Morgan, W.P. (1976). Psychological consequences of vigorous physical activity. In M.G. Scott (Ed.), *The academy papers* (pp. 15-30). Iowa City, IA: American Academy of Physical Education.

Morgan, W.P. (1979a). Anxiety reduction following acute physical activity. *Psychiatric Annals, 9,* 141-147.

Morgan, W.P. (1979b). Negative addiction in runners. *The Physician and Sportsmedicine, 7,* 57-70.

Morgan, W.P. (1979c). Running into addiction. *The Runner, 1,* 72-74.

Morgan, W.P. (1980a). The trait psychology controversy. *Research Quarterly for Exercise and Sport, 51,* 50-76.

Morgan, W.P. (1980b). Sport personology: The credulous-skeptical argument in perspective. In W.F. Straub (Ed.), *Sport psychology: An analysis of athlete behavior* (2nd Ed.). Ithaca, NY: Mouvement Pub.

Morgan, W.P. (1981). Psychological benefits of physical activity. In F.J. Nagle & H.J. Montoye (Eds.), *Exercise, health, and disease.* Springfield, IL: Charles C. Thomas.

Morgan, W.P. (1982). Psychological effects of exercise. *Behavioral Medicine Update, 4,* 25-30.

Morgan, W.P. (1985). Affective beneficience of vigorous physical activity. *Medicine and Science in Sports and Exercise, 17,* 94-100.

Morgan, W.P. (1988). Exercise and mental health. In R.K. Dishman (Ed.), *Exercise adherence: Its impact on public health* (pp. 91-121). Champaign, IL: Human Kinetics.

Morgan, W.P., Brown, D.R., Raglin, J.S., O'Connor, P.J., & Ellickson, K.A. (1987). Psychological monitoring of overtraining and staleness. *British Journal of Sports Medicine, 21,* 107-114.

Morgan, W.P., Costill, D.L., Flynn, M.G., Raglin, J.S., & O'Connor, P.J. (1988). Mood disturbances following increased training in swimmers. *Medicine and Science in Sports and Exercise, 20,* 408-414.

Morgan, W.P., & Goldston, S.E. (1987). *Exercise and mental health.* Washington, DC: Hemisphere Publishing.

Morgan, W.P., & Hammer, W.M. (1974). Influence of competitive wrestling upon state anxiety. *Medicine and Science in Sports and Exercise, 6,* 58.

Morgan, W.P., & Horstman, D.H. (1976). Anxiety reduction following acute physical activity. *Medicine and Science in Sports, 8,* 62.

Morgan, W.P., & O'Connor, P.J. (1988). Exercise and mental health. In R.K. Dishman (Ed.), *Exercise adherence: Its impact on public health* (pp. 91-121). Champaign, IL: Human Kinetics.

Morgan, W.P., & O'Connor, P.J. (1989). Psychological effects of exercise and sports. In E. Ryan & R. Allman (Eds.), *Sports medicine,* (pp. 671-689). New York: Academic Press.

Morgan, W.P., & Pollock, M.L. (1978). Physical activity and cardiovascular health: Psychological aspects. In F. Landry & A. Orban (Eds.), *Physical activity and human well-being* (pp. 163-181). Miami: Symposium Specialists.

Morgan, W.P., Roberts, J.A., Brand, F., & Feinerman, A.O. (1970). Psychological effect of chronic physical activity. *Medicine and Science in Sports, 2,* 213-217.

Morgan, W.P., Roberts, J.A., & Feinerman, A.D. (1971). Psychologic effect of acute physical activity. *Archives of Physical Medicine and Rehabilitation, 52,* 422-425.

Morris, L.W., Davis, M.A., & Hutchins, C.H. (1981). Cognitive and emotional components of anxiety: Literature review and a revised worry-emotionality scale. *Journal of Educational Psychology, 73,* 541-555.

Moses, J., Steptoe, A., Mathews, A., & Edwards, S. (1989). The effects of exercise training on mental well-being in the normal population: A controlled trial. *Journal of Psychosomatic Research, 33*, 47-61.

Mullen, K.D. (1986). *Connections for health*. Dubuque, IA: Wm. C. Brown.

Mutrie, N. (1986). Exercise and treatment for depression within a National Health Service (Doctoral dissertation, Penn State University, 1986). *Dissertation Abstracts International, 47*, 1236A.

Naughton, J., Bruhn, J., & Lategola, M. (1968). Effects of physical training on physiologic and behavioral characteristics of cardiac patients. *Archives of Physical Medicine and Rehabilitation, 49*, 131-137.

Neal, R. (1977). Effect of group counseling and physical fitness programs on self-esteem and cardiovascular fitness (Doctoral dissertation, Boston University, 1977). *Dissertation Abstracts International, 38*, 1911A-1912A.

North, T.C., McCullagh, P., & Tran, Z.V. (1990). Effects of exercise on depression. *Exercise and Sport Science Reviews, 18*, 379-415.

Norvell, N., & Belles, D. (1993). Psychological and physical benefits of circuit weight training in law enforcement personnel. *Journal of Consulting and Clinical Psychology, 61*, 520-527.

Nouri, S., & Beer, J. (1989). Relations of moderate physical exercise to scores on hostility, aggression, and trait anxiety. *Perceptual and Motor Skills, 68*, 1191-1194.

Nowlis, V. (1965). Research with the mood adjective checklist. In S.S. Tomkins & C.E. Izard (Eds.), *Affect, cognition, and personality* (pp. 125-143). New York: Springer.

O'Connor, P.J., Bryant, C.X., Veltri, J.P., & Gebhardt, S.M. (1993). State anxiety and ambulatory blood pressure following resistance exercise in females. *Medicine and Science in Sports and Exercise, 25*, 516-521.

O'Connor, P.J., Carda, R.D., & Graf, B.K. (1991). Anxiety and intense running exercise in the presence and absence of interpersonal competition. *International Journal of Sport Medicine, 12*, 423-426.

Oldridge, N.B. (1982). Compliance and exercise in primary and secondary prevention of coronary heart disease: A review. *Preventive Medicine, 11*, 56-70.

Ossip-Klein, D.J., Doyne, E.J., Bowman, E.D., Osborn, K.M., McDougall-Wilson, J.B., & Neimeyer, R.A. (1989). Effects of running or weight lifting on self-concept in clinically depressed women. *Journal of Consulting and Clinical Psychology, 57*, 158-161.

Otto, J. (1990). The effects of physical exercise on psychophysiological reactions under stress. *Cognition and Emotion, 4*, 341-357.

Palmer, J.H. (1985). Some psychological and physiological effects of aerobic exercise on adult inpatient alcoholics (Doctoral dissertation, University of North Carolina at Greensboro, 1985). *Dissertation Abstracts International, 45*, 1125B.

Panksepp, J. (1986). The neurochemistry of behavior. *Annual Review of Psychology, 37*, 77-107.

Pappas, G.A., Golin, S., & Meyer, D.L. (1990). Reducing symptoms of depression with exercise. *Psychosomatics, 31*, 112-113.

Peele, S. (1981). *How much is too much?* Englewood Cliffs, NJ: Prentice-Hall.

Pelham, T.W., & Campagna, P.D. (1991). Benefits of exercise in psychiatric rehabilitation of persons with schizophrenia. *Canadian Journal of Rehabilitation, 4*, 159-168.

Perls, F., Hefferline, R., & Goodman, P. (1958). *Gestalt therapy.* New York: Julian Press.

Pert, C.B., & Bowie, D.L. (1979). Behavioral manipulation of rats cause alterations in opiate receptor occupancy. In E. Usdin, W.E. Bunney, & N.S. Kline (Eds.), *Endorphins and mental health* (pp. 93-104). New York: Oxford University Press.

Petruzzello, S.J., Landers, D.M., Hatfield, B.D., Kubitz, K.A., & Salazar, W. (1991). A meta-analysis on the anxiety-reducing effects of acute and chronic exercise: Outcomes and mechanisms. *Sports Medicine, 11*, 143-182.

Peyrin, L., & Pequignot, J.M. (1983). Free and conjugated 3-methoxy-4-hydroxyphenyl glycol in human urine: Peripheral origin of the glucuronide. *Psychopharmacology, 79*, 16-20.

Pierce, D., Kupprat, I., & Harry, D. (1976). Urinary epinephrine and norepinephrine levels in women athletes training and competition. *European Journal of Applied Physiology, 36*, 1-6.

Pierce, T.W., Madden, D.J., Siegel, W.C., & Blumenthal, J.A. (1993). Effects of aerobic exercise on cognitive and psychosocial functions in patients with mild hypertension. *Health Psychology, 12*, 286-291.

Pilisuk, M. (1963). Anxiety, self-acceptance, and open-mindedness. *Journal of Clinical Psychology, 19*, 387-391.

Pitts, F.N., & McClure, J.N. (1967). Lactate metabolism in anxiety neurosis. *New England Journal of Medicine, 277*, 1329-1336.

Plummer, O.K., & Koh, V.O. (1987). Effect of "aerobics" on self-concept of college women. *Perceptual and Motor Skills, 65,* 271-275.

Pollock, M.L. (1973). *Exercise and Sports Sciences Review, 1,* 155.

Post, R.M., Kotin, J., & Goodwin, F.K. (1973). Psychomotor activity and cerebrospinal fluid amine metabolites in affective illness. *American Journal of Psychiatry, 130,* 67-72.

Powell, K.E., Spain, K.G., Christenson, G.M., & Mollenkamp, M.P. (1986). The status of the 1990 objectives for physical fitness and exercise. *Public Health Reports, 101,* 15-21.

Prochaska, J.O., Crime, P., Lapandski, D., Martel, L., & Reid, P. (1982). Self-change processes, self-efficacy and self-concept in relapse and maintenance of cessation of smoking. *Psychological Reports, 51,* 983-990.

Radell, S.A., Adame, D.D., & Johnson, T.C. (1993). Dance experiences associated with body-image and personality among college students: A comparison of dancers and nondancers. *Perceptual and Motor Skills, 77,* 507-513.

Raglin, J.S. (1990). Exercise and mental health: Beneficial and detrimental effects. *Sports Medicine, 9,* 323-329.

Raglin, J.S. (1993). Overtraining and staleness: Psychometric monitoring of endurance athletes. In R.N. Singer, M. Murphy, & L.K. Tennant (Eds.), *Handbook of research on sport psychology* (pp. 840-850). New York: Macmillan.

Raglin, J.S., & Morgan, W.P. (1985). Influence of vigorous exercise on mood state. *Behavior Therapist, 8,* 179-183.

Raglin, J.S., & Morgan, W.P. (1987). Influence of exercise and quiet rest on state anxiety and blood pressure. *Medicine and Science in Sports and Exercise, 19,* 456-463.

Raglin, J.S., Turner, P.E., & Eksten, F. (1993). State anxiety and blood pressure following 30 min of leg ergometry or weight training. *Medicine and Science in Sports and Exercise, 25,* 1044-1048.

Ransford, C.P. (1982). A role for amines in the antidepressant effect of exercise: A review. *Medicine and Science in Sports and Exercise, 14,* 1-10.

Regier, D.A., Boyd, J.H., Burke, J.D., Rae, D.S., & Myers, J.K. (1988). One-month prevalence of mental disorders in the United States. *Archives of General Psychiatry, 45,* 977-986.

Regier, D.A., Myers, J.K., Kramer, M., Robins, L.N., Blazer, D.G., Hough, R.L., Eaton, W.W., & Locke, B.Z. (1984). The NIMH epidemiologic catchment area program. *Archives of General Psychiatry, 41,* 934-941.

Rejeski, W.J., Best, D., Griffith, P., & Kenney, E. (1987). Sex-role orientation and the responses of men to exercise stress. *Research Quarterly, 58,* 260-264.

Rejeski, W.J., Hardy, C.J., & Shaw, J. (1991). Psychometric confounds of assessing state anxiety in conjunction with acute bouts of vigorous exercise. *Journal of Sport and Exercise Psychology, 13,* 65-74.

Rejeski, W.J., & Kenney, E.A. (1988). *Fitness motivation: Preventing participant drop-out.* Champaign, IL: Life Enhancement Pub.

Renfrew, N.E., & Bolton, B. (1979). Personality characteristics associated with aerobic exercise in adult males. *Journal of Personality Assessment, 43,* 261-266.

Riggs, C.E. (1981). Endorphins, neurotransmitters and/or neuromodulators and exercise. In M.H. Sacks & M.L. Sachs (Eds.), *Psychology of running* (pp. 224-230). Champaign, IL: Human Kinetics.

Robbins, J.M., & Joseph, P. (1985). Experiencing exercise withdrawal: Possible consequences of therapeutic and mastery running. *Journal of Sport Psychology, 7,* 23-29.

Robins, L.N., Helzer, J.E., Weissman, M.M., Orvaschel, H., Gruenberg, E., Burke, J.D., & Regier, D.A. (1984). Lifetime prevalence of specific psychiatric disorders in three sites. *Archives of General Psychiatry, 41,* 949-958.

Rogers, C.R. (1950). The significance of the self-regarding attitudes and perceptions. In M.L. Reymert (Ed.), *Feeling and emotion: The Moosehart Symposium* (pp. 155-182). New York: McGraw-Hill.

Rosenberg, M. (1965). *Society and the adolescent self-image.* Princeton, NJ: Princeton University Press.

Rosenberg, M. (1979). *Conceiving the self.* New York: Basic Books.

Roskies, E.P., Seraganian, P., Oseasohn, R., Hanley, J.A., Collu, R., Martin, N., & Smilga, C. (1986). The Montreal Type A intervention project: Major findings. *Health Psychology, 5,* 45-69.

Rossier, J., Bloom, F.E., & Guillemin, R. (1980). Endorphins and stress. In H. Selye (Ed.), *Selye's guide to stress research* (Vol. 1, pp. 187-205). New York: VanNostrand Reinhold.

Roth, D.L. (1989). Acute emotional and psychophysiological effects of aerobic exercise. *Psychophysiology, 26,* 593-602.

Roth, D.L., Bachtler, S.D., & Fillingim, R.B. (1990). Acute emotional and cardiovascular effects of stressful mental work during aerobic exercise. *Psychophysiology, 27,* 694-701.

Roth, D.L, & Holmes, D.S. (1987). Influence of aerobic exercise training and relaxation training on physical and psychologic health following stressful life events. *Psychosomatic Medicine, 49,* 355-365.

Roth, W.T. (1974). Some motivational aspects of exercise. *Journal of Sports Medicine and Physical Fitness, 14,* 40-47.

Rotter, J. (1954). *Social learning and clinical psychology.* Englewood Cliffs, NJ: Prentice-Hall.

Rotter, J.B., Chance, J.E., & Phares, E.J. (1972). *Applications of a social learning theory of personality.* New York: Holt, Rinehart & Winston.

Runyan, W.M. (1983). Idiographic goals and methods in the study of lives. *Journal of Personality, 51,* 413-437.

Rushall, B.S. (1972). Three studies relating personality variables to football performance. *International Journal of Sport Psychology, 3,* 12-24.

Rushall, B.S. (1973). The status of personality research and application in sports and physical education. *Journal of Sports Medicine and Physical Fitness, 13,* 281-290.

Rushall, B.S. (1975). Alternative dependent variables for the study of behavior in sport. In D.M. Landers, D.V. Harris, & R.W. Christina (Eds.), *Psychology of sport and motor behavior 2* (pp. 49-55). State College, PA: Pennsylvania State University.

Rushall, B.S. (1978). Environment specific behavior inventories: Developmental procedures. *International Journal of Sport Psychology, 9,* 97-110.

Ryan, A.J. (1983). Overtraining of athletes: A round table. *Physician and Sportsmedicine, 11,* 93-110.

Ryan, A.J. (1984). Exercise and health: Lessons from the past. In M.H. Eckert & H.J. Montoye (Eds.), *Exercise and Health: American Academy of Physical Education papers, 17* (pp. 3-13). Champaign, IL: Human Kinetics.

Sachs, M.L. (1980). *On the trail of the runner's high - A descriptive and experimental investigation of characteristics of an elusive phenomenon.* Unpublished doctoral dissertation, Florida State University, Tallahassee.

Sachs, M.L. (1981). Running addiction. In M.H. Sacks & M.L. Sachs (Eds.), *Psychology of running* (pp. 116-126). Champaign, IL: Human Kinetics.

Sachs, M.L. (1984a). The runner's high. In M.L. Sachs & G.W. Buffone (Eds.), *Running as therapy: An integrated approach* (pp. 55-88). Lincoln, NE: University of Nebraska Press.

Sachs, M.L. (1984b). Psychological well-being and vigorous physical activity. In J.M. Silva & R.S. Weinberg (Eds.), *Psychological foundations of sport* (pp. 435-444). Champaign, IL: Human Kinetics.

Sachs, M.L., & Buffone, G.W. (1984). *Running as therapy: An integrated approach* (Eds.). Lincoln, NE: University of Nebraska Press.

Sacks, M.H., & Sachs, M.L. (1981). *Psychology of running* (Eds.). Champaign, IL: Human Kinetics.

Saipe, M.G. (1978). A morphological investigation of physiological-psychological change (Doctoral dissertation, California School of Professional Psychology, 1977). *Dissertation Abstracts International, 38,* 3905B.

Sanstead, M.J. (1984). The treatment of depression through a graduated aerobic exercise intervention (Doctoral dissertation, University of Nebraska, 1983). *Dissertation Abstracts International, 44,* 2568B.

Sarason, I.G., & Spielberger, C.D. (1976a). *Stress and anxiety* (Vol. 2). New York: John Wiley.

Sarason, I.G., & Spielberger, C.D. (1976b). *Stress and anxiety* (Vol. 3). New York: John Wiley.

Sarason, I.G., & Spielberger, C.D. (1979). *Stress and anxiety.* (Vol. 6). New York: John Wiley.

Schwartz, G.E., Davidson, R.J., & Goleman, D. (1978). Patterning of cognitive and somatic process in the self-regulation of anxiety: Effects of meditation versus exercise. *Psychosomatic Medicine, 40,* 321-328.

Scott, K.A., & Meyers, A.M. (1988). Impact of fitness training on native adolescents' self-evaluations and substance use. *Canadian Journal of Public Health, 79,* 424-429.

Seals, D.R., & Hagberg, J.M. (1984). The effect of exercise training on human hypertension: A review. *Medicine and Science in Sports and Exercise, 16,* 207-215.

Secord, P.F., & Jourard, S.M. (1953). The appraisal of body cathexis: Body cathexis and the self. *Journal of Consulting Psychology, 17,* 343-347.

Seeman, J.C. (1987). Commitment to running, exercise setting, and anxiety reduction (Doctoral dissertation, University of Toledo, 1986). *Dissertation Abstracts International, 47,* 4320A.

Selye, H. (1974). *Stress without distress.* Philadelphia: Lippincott.

Setaro, J.L. (1986). Aerobic exercise and group counseling in the treatment of anxiety and depression (Doctoral dissertation, University of Maryland, 1985). *Dissertation Abstracts International, 47,* 2633B.

Sexton, H., Maere, A., & Dahl, N. (1989). Exercise intensity and reduction in neurotic symptoms: A controlled study. *Acta-Psychiatrica-Scandinavia, 80*, 231-235.

Sforzo, G.A. (1988). Opioids and exercise: An update. *Sports Medicine, 7*, 109-124.

Shapiro, S., Skinner, E.A., Dessler, L.G., VonKorff, M., German, P.S., Tischler, G.L., Leaf, P.J., Benham, L., Cottler, L., & Regier, D.A. (1984). Utilization of health and mental health services. *Archives of General Psychiatry, 41*, 971-978.

Sharkey, B.J. (1974). *Physiological fitness and weight control.* Missoula, MT: Mountain Press Publishing.

Sharkey, B.J. (1979). *Physiology of fitness.* Champaign, IL: Human Kinetics.

Sharp, M.W., & Reilly, R.R. (1975). The relationship of aerobic fitness to selected personality traits. *Journal of Clinical Psychology, 31*, 428-430.

Shavelson, R.J., Hubner, J.J., & Stanton, G.C. (1976). Self-concept: Validation of construct interpretations. *Review of Educational Research, 46*, 407-441.

Sheehan, G. (1983). The best therapy. *The Physician and Sportsmedicine, 11*, 43.

Shepel, L.F. (1984). Depression in social context. In D.P. Lumsden (Ed.), *Community mental health action* (pp. 223-235). Ottawa: Canadian Public Health Association.

Shephard, R.J. (1981). *Ischaemic heart disease and physical activity.* Chicago: Year Book Pub.

Shephard, R.J. (1984). Can we identify those for whom exercise is hazardous? *Sports Medicine, 1*, 75-86.

Shephard, R.J. (1994). *Aerobic fitness & health.* Champaign, IL: Human Kinetics.

Shephard, R.J., Kavanaugh, T., & Klavora, P. (1985). Mood state during postcoronary cardiac rehabilitation. *Journal of Cardiopulmonary Rehabilitation, 5*, 480-484.

Shephard, R.J., & Leith, L.M. (1990). Physical activity and cognitive changes with aging. In M.L. Howe, M.J. Stones, & C.J. Brainerd (Eds.), *Cognitive and behavioral performance factors in atypical aging* (pp. 153-180). New York: Springer-Verlag.

Shorkey, C.T. (1980). Sense of personal worth, self-esteem, and anomie of child abusing mothers and controls. *Journal of Clinical Psychology, 36*, 817-820.

Sime, W.E. (1977). A comparison of exercise and meditation in reducing physiological response to stress. *Medicine and Science in Sports and Exercise, 9*, 55.

Sime, W. (1984). Psychological benefits of exercise training in the healthy individual. In J.D. Matarazzo, S.M. Weiss, J.A. Herd, & N.E. Miller (Eds.), *Behavioral health: A handbook of health enhancement and disease prevention* (pp. 488-508). New York: Wiley Interscience.

Sime, W.E. (1990). Discussion: Exercise, fitness, and mental health. In R. Bouchard, R. Shephard, T. Stephens, J. Sutton, & B. McPherson (Eds.). *Exercise, fitness, and health* (pp. 627-633). Champaign, IL: Human Kinetics.

Simon, G., & Silverman, H. (1990). *The pill book.* New York: Bantam.

Simons, A.D., Epstein, L.H., McGowan, C.R., Kupfer, D.J., & Robertson, R.J. (1985). Exercise as a treatment for depression: An update. *Clinical Psychology Review, 5*, 553-568.

Simons, C.W., & Birkimer, J.C. (1988). An exploration of factors predicting the effect of aerobic conditioning on mood state. *Journal of Psychosomatic Research, 32*, 63-75.

Singer, R.N., Murphy, M., & Tennant, L.K. (1993). *Handbook of research on sport psychology.* New York: Macmillan.

Sinyor, D., Golden, M., Steinert, Y., & Seraganian, P. (1986). Experimental manipulation of aerobic fitness and the response to psychosocial stress: Heart rate and self-report measures. *Psychosomatic Medicine, 48*, 324-337.

Sinyor, D., Schwartz, S.G., Peronnet, F., Brisson, G., & Seraganian, P. (1983). Aerobic fitness level and reactivity to psychosocial stress: Physiological, biochemical, and subjective measures. *Psychosomatic Medicine, 45*, 205-217.

Smith, M., & Glass, G. (1977). Meta-analysis of psychotherapy outcome studies. *American Psychologist, 32*, 995-1008.

Smith, T.P. (1984). An evaluation of the psychological effects of physical exercise on children (Doctoral dissertation, DePaul University, 1983). *Dissertation Abstracts International, 44*, 3260B.

Snyder, S.H. (1977a). The brain's own opiates. *Chemical and Engineering News, 55*, 26-35.

Snyder, S.H. (1977b). Opiate receptors and internal opiates. *Scientific American, 236*, 44-56.

Snyder, S.H. (1980). *Biological aspects of mental disorder.* New York: Oxford University Press.

Solomon, E.G., & Bumpus, A.K. (1978). The running meditation response: An adjunct to psychotherapy. *American Journal of Psychotherapy, 32,* 583-587.

Solomon, R.L. (1980). The opponent-process theory of acquired motivation: The costs of pleasure and the benefits of pain. *American Psychologist, 35,* 691-712.

Solomon, R.L., & Corbit, J.D. (1973). An opponent-process theory of motivation II: Cigarette addiction. *Journal of Abnormal Psychology, 81,* 158-171.

Solomon, R.L., & Corbit, J.D. (1974). An opponent-process theory of motivation I: Temporal dynamics of affect. *Psychological Review, 81,* 119-145.

Soman, V.R., Koivisto, V.A., Deibert, D., Felig, P., & DeFronze, R.A. (1979). Increased insulin sensitivity and insulin bonding to monocytes after physical training. *New England Journal of Medicine, 301,* 1200-1204.

Sonstroem, R.J. (1984). Exercise and self-esteem. In R.L. Terjung (Ed.), *Exercise and sports sciences reviews* (Vol. 12, pp. 123-155). Lexington, MA: Collamore Press.

Sonstroem, R.J., Harlow, L.L., & Josephs, L. (1994). Exercise and self-esteem: Validity of model expansion and exercise associations. *Journal of Sport and Exercise Psychology, 16,* 29-42.

Sonstroem, R.J., Harlow, L.L., & Salisbury, K.S. (1993). Path analysis of a self-esteem model across a competitive swim season. *Research Quarterly for Exercise and Sport, 64,* 335-342.

Sonstroem, R.J. & Morgan, W.P. (1989). Exercise and self-esteem: Rationale and model. *Medicine and Science in Sports and Exercise, 21,* 329-337.

Sothman, M., Horn, T., Hart, B., & Gustafson, A.B. (1987). Comparison of discrete cardiovascular fitness groups on plasma catecholamine and selected behavioral responses to psychological stress. *Psychophysiology, 24,* 47-54.

Sothman, M.S., & Ismail, A.H. (1984). Relationships between urinary catecholamine metabolites, particularly MHPG, and selected personality and physical fitness characteristics in normal subjects. *Psychosomatic Medicine, 46,* 523-533.

Sothman, M.S., & Ismail, A.H. (1985). Factor analytic derivation of the MHPG/NM ratio: Implications for studying the link between physical fitness and depression. *Biological Psychiatry, 20*, 570-583.

Sothman, M.S., Ismail, A.H., & Chodko-Zajko, W.J. (1984). Influence of catecholamine activity on the hierarchical relationships among physical fitness conditions and selected personality characteristics. *Journal of Clinical Psychology, 40*, 1308-1317.

Spielberger, C.D. (1966). Theory and research on anxiety. In C.D. Spielberger (Ed.), *Anxiety and behavior* (pp. 75-104). New York: Academic Press.

Spielberger, C.D. (1972). *Current trends in theory and research* (Vol. 1). New York: Academic Press.

Spielberger, C.D. (1980). *Preliminary manual for the State-Trait Anger Scale (STAS-form X)*. Tampa, FL: University of South Florida Human Resources Institute.

Spielberger, C.D. (1983). *Manual for the state-trait anxiety inventory (Form Y)*. Palo Alto, CA: Consulting Psychologists Press.

Spielberger, C.D., Gorsuch, R.L., & Lushene, R.E. (1970). *The state trait anxiety scale*. Palo Alto, CA: Consulting Psychologists Press.

Spielberger, C.D., & Sarason, I.G. (1975). *Stress and anxiety* (Vol. 1). New York: John Wiley.

Spielberger, C.D., & Sarason, I.G. (1977). *Stress and anxiety* (Vol. 4). New York: John Wiley.

Spielberger, C.D., & Sarason, I.G. (1978). *Stress and anxiety* (Vol. 5). New York: John Wiley.

Spirduso, W.W. (1983). Exercise and the aging brain. *Research Quarterly for Exercise and Sports, 54*, 208-218.

Sports Council (1982). *Sport in the community: The next ten years*. London: The Sports Council.

Steege, J.F., & Blumenthal, J.A. (1993). The effects of aerobic exercise on premenstrual symptoms in middle-aged women: A preliminary study. *Journal of Psychosomatic Research, 37*, 127-133.

Stein, P.N., & Motta, R.W. (1992). Effects of aerobic and nonaerobic exercise on depression and self-concept. *Perceptual and Motor Skills, 74*, 79-89.

Steinberg, H., & Sykes, E.A. (1985). Introduction to symposium on endorphins and behavioral processes: Review of literature on endorphins and exercise. *Pharmacology Biochemistry and Behavior, 23*, 857-862.

Stephens, T. (1988). Physical and mental health in the United States and Canada: Evidence from four population surveys. *Preventive Medicine, 17*, 35-47.

Steptoe, A., Edwards, S., Moses, J., & Mathews, A. (1989). The effects of exercise training on mood and perceived coping ability in anxious adults from the general population. *Journal of Psychosomatic Research, 33*, 537-547.

Steptoe, A., & Kearsley, N. (1990). Cognitive and somatic anxiety. *Behavior Research and Therapy, 28*, 75-81.

Steptoe, A., Moses, J., Edwards, S., & Mathews, A. (1993). Exercise and responsivity to mental stress: Discrepancies between the subjective and physiological effects of aerobic training. *International Journal of Sport Psychology, 24*, 110-129.

Stern, J.J., & Cleary, P.J. (1982). The National Exercise and Heart Disease Project: Long term psychosocial outcomes. *Archives of Internal Medicine, 142*, 1093-1097.

Stern, P., Chilnick, L.D., Simon, G.I., & Silverman, H.M. (1990). *The pill book.* New York: Bantam Books.

Stone, M.H., O'Bryant, H., & Garhammer, J. (1981). A hypothetical model for strength training. *Journal of Sports Medicine and Physical Fitness, 21*, 342-351.

Sweeney, D.R., Leckman, J.F., Maas, J.W., Hattox, S., & Heninger, G.R. (1980). Plasma free and conjugated MHPG in psychiatric patients. *Archives of General Psychiatry, 37*, 1100-1103.

Sweeney, D.R., Maas, J.W., & Heninger, G.R. (1978). State anxiety, physical activity and urinary 3-methoxy-4-hydroxyphenethylene glycol excretion. *Archives of General Psychiatry, 35*, 1418-1425.

Tang, S.W., Stancer, H.C., Takahashi, S., Shephard, R.J., & Warsh, J.J. (1981). Controlled exercise elevates plasma but not urinary MHPG and VMA. *Psychiatry Research, 4*, 13-20.

Taxe, P.W. (1985). An exploratory investigation in the use of aerobic exercise as a stress management technique in short-term therapy (Doctoral dissertation, United States International University, 1978). *Dissertation Abstracts International, 46*, 1348B.

Taylor, C.B., Houston-Miller, N., Ahn, D.K., Haskell, W., & DeBusk, R.F. (1986). The effects of exercise training programs on psychosocial improvement in uncomplicated postmyocardial incarction patients. *Journal of Psychosomatic Research, 30*, 581-587.

Taylor, J.A. (1953). A personality scale of manifest anxiety. *Journal of Abnormal and Social Psychology, 48,* 285-290.

Tenario, L.M. (1986). Effects of aerobic exercise on symptoms of depression in women (Doctoral dissertation, Texas Women's University, 1986). *Dissertation Abstracts International, 47,* 2367B.

Tharp, G.D., & Carson, W.H. (1975). Emotionality changes in rats following chronic exercise. *Medicine and Science in Sports and Exercise, 7,* 123-126.

Thayer, R.E. (1985). Activation (arousal): The shift from a single to multidimensional perspective. In J. Strelau, T. Gale, & F. Farley (Eds.), *The biological basis of personality and behavior* (pp. 115-127). Washington DC: Hemisphere.

Thayer, R.E. (1987). Energy, tiredness, and tension effects of a sugar snack versus moderate exercise. *Journal of Personality and Social Psychology, 52,* 119-125.

Thompson, J.K., & Marten, J.E. (1984). Exercise in health modification: Assessment and training guidelines. *Behavior Therapist, 7,* 5-8.

Thoren, P., Floras, J.S., Hoffman, P., & Seals, D.R. (1990). Endorphins and exercise: Physiological mechanisms and clinical applications. *Medicine and Science in Sports and Exercise, 22,* 417-428.

Tillman, K. (1965). Relationship between physical fitness and selected personality traits. *Research Quarterly, 36,* 483-489.

Topp, R. (1989). Effect of relaxation or exercise on undergraduate test anxiety. *Perceptual and Motor Skills, 69,* 35-41.

Tucker, L. (1983). Effect of weight training on self-concept: A profile of those influenced most. *Research Quarterly for Exercise and Sports, 54,* 389-397.

Tucker, L.A. (1982a). Effect of a weight-training program on the self-concept of college males. *Perceptual and Motor Skills, 54,* 1055-1061.

Tucker, L.A. (1982b). Relationship between perceived somatotype and body cathexis of college males. *Psychological Reports, 50,* 983-989.

Valliant, P.M., & Asu, M.E. (1985). Exercise and its effect on cognition and physiology in older adults. *Perceptual and Motor Skills, 61,* 1031-1038.

Van Loon, G.R., Schwartz, L., & Sole, M.J. (1979). Plasma dopamine responses to standing and exercise in man. *Life Sciences, 24,* 2273-2278.

Veale, D.M.W. (1991). Psychological aspects of staleness and dependence on exercise. *International Journal of Sports Medicine, 12,* 19-22.

Verstraeten, D. (1987). Personality research and the measurement of change: A review over twenty years. *Tijdschrift voor Klinische Psychologie, 17,* 232-253.

Villet, B. (1978). Opiates of the mind. *The Atlantic, 241,* 82-89.

Wang, Y., & Morgan, W.P. (1987). Convergent validity of a body awareness scale. *Medicine and Science in Sports and Exercise, 19,* S579.

Wardlaw, S.L., & Frantz, A.G. (1980). Effect of swimming stress on brain B-endorphin and ACTH (Abstract). *Clinical Research, 28,* 482.

Watkins, D., & Park, J. (1972). The role of subjective importance in self-evaluation. *Australian Journal of Psychology, 24,* 209-210.

Watson, D., Clark, L.A., & Tellegen, A. (1988). Development and validation of brief measures of positive and negative affect: The PANAS scales. *Journal of Personality and Social Psychology, 54,* 1063-1070.

Weaver, D.C. (1985). A study to determine the effect of exercise on depression in middle-aged women (Doctoral dissertation, Tennessee State University, 1984). *Dissertation Abstracts International, 45,* 2033A.

Weber, J.C., & Lee, R.A. (1968). Effects of differing prepuberty exercise programs on the emotionality of male albino rats. *Research Quarterly, 39,* 748-751.

Weinberg, R., Jackson, A., & Kolodny, K. (1988). The relationship of massage and exercise to mood enhancement. *The Sport Psychologist, 2,* 202-211.

Weinberg, R.S., Hughes, H.H., Critelli, J.W., England, R., & Jackson, A. (1984). Effects of preexisting and manipulated self-efficacy on weight loss in a self-control program. *Journal of Research in Personality, 18,* 352-358.

Weiss, J., Singh, M., & Youdal, L. (1983). Occipital and parietal alpha power before, during, and after exercise (abstract). *Medicine and Science in Sports and Exercise, 15,* 117.

Weiss, J.M. (1982). A model of neurochemical study of depression. Paper presented at the Annual Convention of the American Psychological Association, Washington, D.C.

Werner, A., & Gottheil, E. (1966). Personality development and participation in college athletics. *Research Quarterly, 37,* 126-131.

White, A. (1974). The interrelationships between measures of physical fitness and measures of self-concept of selected Mississippi State University male students (Doctoral dissertation, Mississippi State University, 1973). *Dissertation Abstracts International, 34,* 4849A.

Wicklund, R.A. (1975). Objective self-awareness. In L. Berkowitz (Ed.), *Advances in experimental social psychology* (Vol. 8, pp.456-465). New York: Academic Press.

Wilfley, D., & Kunce, J. (1986). Differential physical and psychological effects of exercise. *Journal of Counseling Psychology, 33,* 337-342.

Williams, J.M., & Getty, D. (1986). Effects of levels of exercise on psychological mood states. *Perceptual and Motor Skills, 63,* 1099-1105.

Wilson, A., & Krane, R. (1980). Change in self-esteem and its effects on symptoms of depression. *Cognitive Therapy Research, 4,* 419-421.

Wilson, V.E., Berger, B.G., & Bird, E.I. (1981). Effect of running and of an exercise class on anxiety. *Perceptual and Motor Skills, 53,* 472-474.

Wilson, V.E., Morley, N.C., & Bird, E.I. (1980). Mood profiles of marathon runners, joggers, and non-exercisers. *Perceptual and Motor Skills, 50,* 117-118.

Wylie, R.C. (1979). *The self-concept: Theory and research on selected topics* (Vol. 2). Lincoln, NE: University of Nebraska Press.

Yates, A., Leehey, K., & Slisslak, C.M. (1983). Running - An analogue of anorexia? *New England Journal of Medicine, 308,* 251-255.

Young, R.J. (1979). The effect of regular exercise on cognitive functioning and personality. *British Journal of Sports Medicine, 13,* 110-117.

Young, R.J., & Ismail, A.H. (1976). Personality differences of adult men before and after a physical fitness program. *Research Quarterly, 47,* 513-519.

Zeiss, L.P., & Munoz, R. (1979). Nonspecific improvement effects in depression using interpersonal skills training, pleasant activity schedules, or cognitive training. *Journal of Consulting and Clinical Psychology, 47,* 427-439.

Zion, L.C. (1965). Body concept as it relates to self-concept. *Research Quarterly, 36,* 490-495.

Zorn, S.M. (1989). The psychological effects of exercise during pregnancy and postpartum (Doctoral dissertation, Temple University, 1988). *Dissertation Abstracts International, 49,* 1962B.

Zuckerman, M., & Lubin, B. (1965). *Manual for the Multiple Affect Adjective Checklist.* San Diego: Educational and Industrial Testing Service.

Zung, W.W. (1965). Self-rating depression scale. *Archives of General Psychiatry, 12,* 63.

SUBJECT INDEX

About the Author

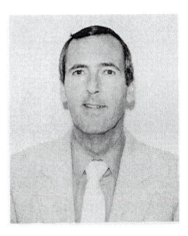

Larry M. Leith is a professor in the Department of Physical and Health Education at the University of Toronto. He holds a cross-appointment with the Department of Behavioral Sciences in the Faculty of Medicine. Dr. Leith teaches undergraduate courses in Sport Psychology, Health Psychology, and Sports Administration. At the graduate level, Larry has designed and implemented a course entitled Exercise Psychology, utilizing many of the concepts covered in this textbook. Dr. Leith has published over 90 articles dealing with health psychology, sport psychology, and other areas of human behavior.

Larry attempts to practice what he preaches by participating in regular jogging and walking programs. His favorite sports are tennis and golf. Larry and his wife Nancy reside in Guelph, Ontario.